THE NATURAL DIABETES CURE

Curing Blood Sugar Disorders Without Drugs

ROGER MASON

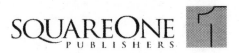

SQUAREONE
PUBLISHERS

The Natural Diabetes Cure is not intended as medical advice. It is written solely for informational and educational purposes. Please consult a health professional should the need for one be indicated. Because there is always some risk involved, the author and publisher are not responsible for any adverse affects or consequences resulting from the use of any of the suggestions, preparations or methods described in the book. The publisher does not advocate the use of any particular diet or health program, but believes the information presented in this book should be available to the public.

All listed addresses, phone numbers and fees have been reviewed and updated during production. However, the data is subject to change.

EDITOR: Erica Shur
TYPESETTER: Gary A. Rosenberg

Square One Publishers
115 Herricks Road
Garden City Park, NY 11040
(516) 535-2010 • (877) 900-BOOK
www.squareonepublishers.com

Library of Congress Cataloging-in-Publication Data

10   9   8   7   6   5   4   3   2   1

Contents

Other Health Books
by Roger Mason

Lower Blood Pressure Without Drugs

Lower Your Cholesterol Without Drugs

Natural Health for Women

The Minerals You Need

The Natural Prostate Cure

No More Horse Estrogen!

Testosterone Is Your Friend

What Is Beta Glucan?

Zen Macrobiotics for Everyone

Introduction

Blood sugar problems can be potentially serious and lead to chronic diseases. When too many simple sugars are taken into the body, by either food or drink, your blood sugar rises. All blood sugar conditions should be treated the same way with diet and lifestyle: a healthy diet, proven supplements, an exercise plan, taking natural hormones, avoiding prescription drugs, weekly fasting (if possible), and avoiding bad habits.

As long as you have an intact pancreas, you can cure yourself. Those whose pancreas has irreversibly atrophied or been surgically removed can still dramatically improve their health and reduce their insulin requirements.

Diabetes and other blood sugar disorders are caused by what we eat and the way we live. You can cure yourself by making healthier food choices and living better. You can heal yourself in less than a year if you are sincere.

Diabetes is the fastest growing epidemic in the Western world. One in three American children will grow up and needlessly develop diabetes. Twenty-four percent of American adults are insulin resistant and 45 percent of adults over the age of sixty are insulin resistant. In the last three decades diabetes and other blood sugar problems have become epidemics in all of the developed countries of the world. It is estimated that about 18 million

Americans have diabetes, 16 million are prediabetic, and a whopping 60 million (one in five) have metabolic syndrome. America leads the world in blood sugar dysmetabolism for a very simple reason; we have the greatest affluence, as well as the worst diets and lifestyles. We are overfed and undernourished.

Changing your diet and lifestyle will both prevent and cure blood sugar disorders. The medical profession cannot help you; you must help yourself. Treating the symptoms with toxic drugs is the road to ruin. You have to be your own doctor and your own saviour. You must be willing to eat better foods, get regular exercise, and change your lifestyle. *The Natural Diabetes Cure* is the most researched, effective, documented, comprehensive, and complete book on diabetes and blood sugar problems available. This research goes back over thirty years. Everything is backed up by countless published international clinical studies.

1. About Diabetes

According to statistics, diabetes is the fastest growing disease in the world. Currently, one in every ten people have diabetes in the United States, and that number is increasing. It is estimated that in two decades, it will be one out of every three people who has this terrible, yet very preventable disease. It is also on the rise in Europe, Australia, India, Japan, and China. By understanding some of the basics of diabetes, you will be in a better position to understand why it is increasing at such a rapid rate, and what you can do either to stop it from happening or reverse it.

Diabetes is classified as a metabolic disorder. Every cell in our body needs energy to function and grow. The several processes by which our body produces this energy is called metabolism. When this process is disrupted or put into a state of imbalance, your health is at great risk. We eat food not only for their many nutrients, but also for the energy that they provide for our body. When food is digested, it is broken down into its individual parts. *Glucose*, a simple sugar, is used to create energy. However, the glucose that is produced cannot enter our cells without the presence of insulin. *Insulin*, a hormone, is produced by the pancreas. The pancreas needs to release an adequate amount of insulin to move the glucose in our blood into our cells to lower our blood sugar level. When the body does not produce enough insulin or produces no insulin, or when the cells do not respond properly to the insulin, a condition in which the amount of glucose in the blood is elevated occurs. This condition is diabetes.

LEADING CAUSES OF DIABETES

Metabolic syndrome, or prediabetes—blood glucose levels that are higher than normal but not yet high enough to be diagnosed as diabetes—is the fastest rising epidemic on the planet. This condition is characterized by obesity, insulin resistance, dyslipidemia (high or low blood fats), hypertension, and high insulin.

Obesity

Obesity means having too much body fat; it is not the same as being overweight. A person may be overweight, which means weighing too much, from extra muscle or water. Sometimes it is a combination of both. Taking in more calories than you can burn leads to obesity, and it may be responsible for 75 percent of the problem.

Insulin Resistance

Insulin resistance is a condition in which the body produces insulin. However, the body doesn't always use it properly. When a person is insulin resistant, their body doesn't respond properly to insulin, and their body needs more insulin to help the glucose enter their cells. The pancreas tries to keep up with this demand, but eventually fails to. This condition most often goes undiagnosed. People may have this condition for several years without noticing anything.

Hypertension

Hypertension is another epidemic. It is a term medical practitioners use to describe high blood pressure. Blood pressure is the force of the blood flow inside your blood vessels. Your blood pressure is recorded as two numbers (a top and a bottom), and both numbers are important. The first number is the pressure as your heart beats and pushes the blood through the blood vessels; it is referred to as the *systolic pressure*. The second number is the pressure when the vessels are relaxed between heartbeats; this is referred to as the *diastolic pressure*. Your blood pressure is high when your blood moves through your vessels with too much force. Hypertension is a condition characterized by chronically high blood pressure. Seventy-five percent of people who suffer from hypertension have diabetes. Hypertension is an important risk factor for the development and the worsening of diabetes.

Dyslipidemia

Dyslipidemia is the condition of having too high or too low levels of fats (lipids) in the bloodstream. Cholesterol and triglycerides are the fatty substances produced by the body, and they are known as lipids. Fat cells respond to insulin and the effect is a decrease in the levels of fatty acids in the blood. When one suffers from diabetes there is a deficiency of insulin released into the blood, which leads to dyslipidemia. High blood cholesterol, and especially triglycerides, is a concern for people suffering from diabetes. Diabetes is associated with a high risk of coronary disease; therefore, dyslipidemia is a risk factor that should be identified early.

High Blood Insulin

High blood insulin levels also go undiagnosed. Insulin is a hormone that causes most of the body's cells to take up glucose (sugars) from the blood. If you have too much sugar in your blood vessels, it is likely that you also have too much insulin in your bloodstream. When you eat sugary foods, glucose is released into your bloodstream. Insulin works by stimulating your cells to absorb the excess sugar out of your bloodstream. If you eat too many sugary foods and too many processed carbohydrates, your body will release so much insulin that the cells won't receive as strong a signal to absorb the excess sugar from the blood. This condition leads to diabetes and other chronic conditions.

FASTEST GROWING DISEASE

Diabetes is the most serious and deadly condition. Currently, this is the fifth leading cause of death in the United States, and will soon be the fourth leading cause. Almost twenty million Americans now have actual diabetes, which means about one in every fifteen. In addition, there are probably about six million more, mostly poor people, who have diabetes and simply haven't been medically diagnosed. A million more are newly diagnosed every year. These are mostly the impoverished and elderly, who can't afford the medical care they need. All in all, this would mean about one in twelve Americans are diabetic, with the rates rising every year! This is the fastest growing disease of all worldwide. India and China are also coping with growing epidemics. In the 1990s, the diabetes rate in America increased a full one-third. Almost $150 billion a year is spent directly and indirectly worldwide on diabetes treatment. This money is basically wasted on toxic, harmful prescription drugs such as metformin, Januvia, Onglyza, Amaryl, Avandia, Glucotrol, and Actos. None of these drug therapies are effective; actually, they worsen your health.

METABOLIC SYNDROME

Metabolic syndrome, or Syndrome X, is a cluster of the most dangerous factors that increase the risk of diabetes, coronary heart disease, and stroke. Elevated blood glucose levels, high blood pressure, obesity, and abnormal blood lipid levels are conditions that tend to occur together in certain people and lead to metabolic syndrome. Age and race are also factors to be considered. The risk of metabolic syndrome increases as you get older, and there is a greater risk of metabolic syndrome among Asians and Hispanics.

About one in four American adults suffer from metabolic syndrome and will soon be diagnosed with diabetes. Half of all diabetes goes undiagnosed! According to the Center for Disease Control (CDC) in Atlanta, one in three children born today in the United States will develop type 2 diabetes. One in three American children will be diabetic! Age is one of the biggest factors, since one in four Americans over the age of 65 are diabetic. Stress is also an important factor, and most Westerners are under a good deal of self-imposed stress. No other country in the world will approach these statistics. Blacks, Latins, Asians, and Amerindians suffer disproportionately. American Pima Indians, for example, have almost a 50-percent rate of outright diabetes. Mexican Pima Indians, on the other hand, follow their traditional diet and lifestyle. They have a very low rate of just a few percent. One-fourth of adult Navajo Indians are diabetic, according to CDC statistics. Asian adults in America generally have almost a 40 percent rate of diabetes, yet this is rare in the rural areas of Asia. Many Asian cities have now largely adopted the Western high-fat, high-sugar, refined foods diet, and their diabetes rates are soaring. Latin adults in America generally have a 15 percent diabetes rate, but not in their native countries. In Papua, New Guinea—possibly the least civilized country in the world—diabetes is basically unknown. Black American adults now have a high overall 15 percent diabetes rate. Yet, this is rare in Africa, where they eat their traditional diet. Caucasian American adults have the lowest overall rate.

The CDC recently studied 8,814 normal men and women. They found that 22 percent of them exhibited at least three of the six factors of metabolic syndrome. People over sixty, with three of the factors, had a 44 percent rate, or double the average. This means almost half of Americans over the age of sixty are prediabetic.

Prediabetes means that your blood sugar level is higher than normal. This condition is called *prediabetes*, since such people can plan on becoming diabetic within ten years. Again, the basic indications are obesity (especially abdominal), insulin resistance, elevated blood sugar, high cholesterol and triglycerides, and hypertension.

TYPES OF DIABETES

There are three main types of diabetes. *Type 1* (insulin-dependent) *diabetes* is due to the inability of the beta cells in the pancreas to produce insulin. Only 5 percent to 10 percent of people suffer from type 1 diabetes. Surprisingly, Caucasians are more susceptible to this form. This usually happens in childhood or adolescence. These patients have to inject insulin, since they can't produce it naturally. If the pancreas has been removed or is atrophied, the condition cannot be cured. Quality of life can be improved immensely, and insulin requirements can be reduced dramatically by following the advice in this book. Pancreas transplants just don't work, despite the claims. Transplanting a pancreas from a cadaver to a type 1 diabetic requires dangerous anti-rejection drugs and causes countless problems. Transplants of just the pancreatic beta cells also promise much more than is delivered. Within twenty years, science may be able to successfully perform this procedure, but that will merely be allopathic. It will not deal with the cause!

Type 2 diabetes is the most common form of diabetes. Millions of American people have been diagnosed with type 2, and there are many more people who are unaware that they may be at high risk. This type of diabetes is more common in African Americans, Native Americans, Latinos, Asian Americans, as well as older people. It can be a lifelong chronic disease in which there are high levels of sugar or glucose in the blood. Type 2 diabetics (non-insulin-dependent) produce insulin, but the cells simply don't react well to it anymore. Here, the pancreas not only produces insulin, but usually overproduces it, since the effectiveness is so reduced when there is an excessive amount of sugar (glucose) in the bloodstream. This type is very curable, usually within a year or less.

The third type is called *gestational diabetes*, since it only affects pregnant women. Pregnant women who have never had diabetes before their pregnancy, but have high blood sugar (glucose) levels during pregnancy, are diagnosed with gestational diabetes. This condition affects the mother in late pregnancy after the baby's body has been formed. For some reason, women who have gestational diabetes during pregnancy are more susceptible to diabetes in later life.

OXIDATIVE STRESS

The best way to understand the dysfunction of insulin and blood sugar is the theory of *oxidative stress*. Here free radicals run rampant through the body and use up our antioxidants—glutathione, SOD (superoxide dismutase), beta carotene, vitamin E, vitamin C, CoQ_{10}, melatonin, lipoic acid, and others. This is why it is so important, first of all, to lower oxidative stress with better diet and exercise. Secondly, we need to take all the known antioxidant supplements to neutralize the excess free radicals. These supplements are discussed in detail in Chapters 6 and 7. The high rates of alcohol and nicotine use add to oxidative stress. Coffee (or any form of caffeine) raises blood sugar and has other very serious health effects. The scientists of the world are in basic agreement that free radical oxidative stress is central to blood sugar conditions.

CONCLUSION

About half a million Americans die every year from diabetes. If you are diabetic, you have about three times the rate of strokes, about three times the rate of heart attacks, and greatly increased rates of atherosclerosis (clogged arteries). Remember that heart disease is the number one cause of death and the biggest killer by far. Blindness and vision problems are called *diabetic retinopathy*, and are an epidemic for people with impaired blood sugar metabolism. Amputation of limbs due to poor circulation is common. Various cancers, gastrointestinal infections, osteoporosis, erectile dysfunction, poorly healing wounds, kidney infections and failure, and poor sleep are all part and parcel here. Your mental make-up is affected, including depression, senility, Alzheimer's, impaired memory, and other problems. Any blood sugar dysfunction means poor quality of life and early death. The pancreas deteriorates, nerve damage of various kinds can be expected, liver disease is routine, and skin infections (especially *Staphylococcus*) are common. Your liver is central here, since it produces the blood sugar from the food you eat. Your kidneys are the second most important organs. The list of side effects is almost endless, since the total health of the body is destroyed.

If you have type 1 diabetes, pancreas transplants and beta cell (the insulin-producing pancreatic cells) transplants just don't work at all. You can dramatically reduce your insulin requirements, reduce your medication, and improve your health immensely with the information in this book. Even if your pancreas has been removed or atrophied beyond repair, you can still live a good life with minimal insulin. Anyone with type 2 diabetes can cure themselves within a year and live a normal, healthy life.

2. Diagnosis

Identifying risk factors for diabetes is crucial. Unknown millions of Americans of all ages have prediabetes. This is especially true for those over forty. It is estimated that one-third of outright diabetics just aren't aware that they have diabetes. This is especially true for the poor and less educated. Prediabetes tends to lead to actual full-blown diabetes. This certainly can be prevented and reversed with diet and lifestyle. The major risk factors are obesity, hypertension, insulin resistance, low HDL cholesterol, high LDL cholesterol, high triglycerides, high homocysteine, elevated uric acid, increased C-reactive protein, hypercoagulability of the blood, fasting blood glucose over 85 milligrams per deciliter (mg/dL) (European mmol is 4.7), HbA1c over 4.7 per cent, low white blood cell count, high creatinine, and albuminuria (albumin protein in the urine). Age is critical as well. The older you are, the more blood sugar problems you can expect. Diabetes rates go up dramatically among people over the age of fifty. Genetics is not that vital, even though a family history of diabetes does raise your chances. Obesity is one of the cornerstone factors, and an entire chapter has been devoted to it. Race is very important. You are far more at risk if you are of African, Asian, Amerindian, or Latin origin. Caucasians have the lowest rates (except type 1). Smokers get far more diabetes than others, as do people who drink substantial amounts of alcohol or use caffeine.

DIAGNOSTIC TESTS

An ounce of prevention is worth ten pounds of cure. You must get certain basic diagnostic tests not only to prevent diabetes, but also for your general health. These are basic and inexpensive, and can be done on the Internet without a doctor. Currently, we do not have inexpensive practical tests for total oxidative stress or general free radical activity. It is costly and unnecessary to get exotic tests for antioxidants such as SOD (superoxide dismutase), glutathione, vitamin C, beta carotene, and vitamin E. The antioxidants you should take are discussed in detail in Chapter 6 on supplements (see page 41).

A standard blood analysis should include glucose, total cholesterol, HDL cholesterol, LDL cholesterol, triglycerides, uric acid, C-reactive protein, homocysteine, white blood cell count, and creatinine. It should also include the liver assays SGOT/AST and SGPT/ALT. (These are aspartate aminotransferase and alanine aminotransferase.) You want to be in the lower half of the range for both SGOT and SGPT. You can also ask for an albumin urine test for kidney function. Good kidney function is crucial here. Let's discuss the basic tests you should get.

Glucose Tolerance Test

The most accurate test you can get for insulin resistance is a GTT (glucose tolerance test). This is far more predictive than testing your insulin per se. If your blood sugar level is over 85 mg/dL you need to do this. The GTT shows the sensitivity of your insulin response. It is the Gold Standard, inexpensive, non-invasive, accurate, and safe, but very underutilized for some reason. Simply get a fasting one hour, one blood draw test. (You should already know your fasting blood sugar level.) You drink a 50-g cup of glucose solution, wait one hour, and then see how high your blood sugar has risen. This shows how well your muscles respond to insulin. Use 20 points under the accepted medical level. If their "official" figure is 140 mg/dL, then you want 120 mg/dL.

Fasting Blood Sugar

Your fasting blood sugar is the most obvious test. Look for a level of 85 mg/dL or less (European 4.7 mmol). You can buy inexpensive (about ten dollars) and very accurate blood sugar meters in any chain drugstore. The True series is very good. Doctors will accept any reading under 100 mg/dL as "normal," but this is not true at all. The international research shows that people with sugar levels under 85 mg/dL live longer and are healthier than those with levels over 85 mg/dL. This is especially true with cardiovascular disease (CHD), the biggest killer of all by far worldwide. Keep your blood sugar level under 85 mg/dL. Simple sugars and caffeine will raise it.

Blood Pressure

Blood pressure is basic here, and you should look for a reading of 120/80 or better. Inexpensive home electronic monitors are widely available in drug stores and on the Internet. Remember that hypertension is the most common medical condition on earth and even prominent in agrarian Third World countries. High blood pressure equates to poor health, low quality of life, strokes, and early death.

HbA1c Test

The HbA1c (hemoglobin glycation) test shows long-term *glycation* (sugar molecules attached to hemoglobin) over a six-month period. You want 4.7 percent (equals 85 mg/dL blood sugar) or better here, and not the usual 5.6 percent (equals 100 mg/dL blood sugar) medical standard. This is a good test, but optional. You can get exotic tests such as leptin, malondialdehyde, thrombomodulin, tumor necrosis factor (TNF), adiponectin, plasminogen, fibrinogen, and others. These are expensive, unneeded, and not necessary or practical. Spend your time, energy, attention, and money on curing yourself and changing your diet and lifestyle, rather than getting diagnostics you don't need.

Total Cholesterol and Triglycerides

Your blood lipids total cholesterol (TC) and triglycerides (TG) are all important. These are the two most important CHD diagnostic markers of all. You should also get your HDL and LDL levels done as well. Your TC should ideally be about 150 mg/dL, and not the usual American average of 240 mg/dL. Animal fats are the culprit here. It is not enough to keep this under 200 mg/dL. Even if you have genetically high blood lipids you can keep this at least under 200 mg/dL. Your TG level is the most important blood lipid marker of all regarding blood sugar issues. Keep this under 100 mg/dL. Simple sugars are the culprit here. Even vegans and ethical vegetarians can (and usually do) have high TG levels due to inordinate intake of various sugars. People with blood sugar problems generally have low HDL ("good" cholesterol) and high LDL ("bad" cholesterol). Diet and lifestyle will lower TC, TG, and LDL levels, while raising HDL levels.

C-reactive Protein

C-reactive protein (CRP) is an important inflammation marker for diabetes, as well as CHD of all kinds. Inflammation is characterized by redness, swelling, tenderness, heat, pain, and impaired cell function. Inflammation is an epidemic in developed countries. CRP is an independent risk factor for both type 1 and type 2 diabetes. On a range of 0 to 3 you want to be under 1.0 mg/dL. Now American children commonly have high CRP levels.

High CRP correlates with obesity, high blood glucose, insulin resistance, hypertension, high triglycerides, and uric acid. Everyone over the age of forty should know their CRP level. Even younger people should get theirs tested, since one in three will grow up to develop type 2 diabetes, and CHD is the biggest killer by far worldwide. Diet and lifestyle will dramatically lower CRP very quickly.

Uric Acid

Uric acid (UA) is a proven independent risk factor here. The research is very strong. You can find low uric acid in type 1 diabetics, however, due to excessive excretion of it. High UA in the blood is clearly associated with obesity, high triglycerides, high systolic blood pressure, and a high TC-to-HDL ratio. High UA is especially related to high TG and obesity. Excess uric acid comes from eating the animal proteins in meat, poultry, eggs, and dairy foods. It does not come from purines as commonly thought. The widespread purine theory is simply incorrect. Dairy foods, for example, have almost no purines but still raise UA. High uric acid levels are generally only found in the affluent, developed countries where animal foods are staples. It is also clear that simple sugars raise UA just as they raise triglycerides. It is very possible that one-third of all US adults have hyperuricemia. If the range for men is 3.6 mg/dL to 8.3 mg/dL (214 to 494 mmol), you want to be definitely under 6.0 mg/dL. If the range for women is 2.3 mg/dL to 6.6 mg/dL (137 to 393 mmol), you want to be definitely under 4.5 mg/dL. Just don't eat animal products except for 10-percent seafood. Moderate exercise dramatically lowers UA.

Homocysteine

Homocysteine (Hcys) is also a very accurate marker of both blood sugar disorders and CHD events in general. The levels for type 1 diabetics can actually be lower than normal, however. This shows there are differences in type 1 and type 2. Hcys is a very basic and vital marker for heart and artery health in general. You want to definitely be in the lower half of the given range. Men have higher levels of Hcys. With a range of 6.4 mmol/L to 13.7 mmol/L in men, you should keep your level below 10.0 mmol/L. With a range of 3.4 mmol/L to 12.9 mmol/L in women, you should keep your level below 8.1 mmol/L. This is very easy to do if you eat well.

Creatinine

Creatinine is part of standard blood tests. This is an excellent kidney marker. Your blood levels of creatinine should be at the low end. The kidneys are central to blood sugar metabolism just as the liver is. The secret to good kidney health is a low protein diet. Americans eat twice the protein they need. Kidney disease is an epidemic in America. Your urinary albumin excretion should be in the normal range. Excess protein in your urine is called *microalbuminuria*. You can get inexpensive urine test strips in the drugstore to check this rather than seeing a doctor. These are all the diagnostic tests you need. Put your time, energy, and money into curing yourself with diet and lifestyle.

CONCLUSION

As our attitude towards disease changes, we learn to focus on prevention of chronic diseases such as diabetes. Knowing the risk factors and monitoring them by using diagnostic tests becomes critical in the prevention and management of diabetes. Although an important factor in the development of diabetes is genetics, there are things in our environment that we can learn to control in order to lower the risk of developing diabetes, or curing blood sugar disorders without drugs. Once again, we must make diet, exercise, and a healthy lifestyle a priority.

3. Whole Grains— The Staff of Life

Whole grains are literally "the staff of life," and have been the staple food of almost all civilizations throughout history. Since man started agriculture about 10,000 years ago, whole grains have been the principal food of most people in the world. Rice and wheat are the most consumed foods on earth. This emancipated us from being mere primitive hunters and gatherers. The Paleolithic people, on this Stone Age diet of wild plants and animals, had very short life spans. The cultivation of whole grains parallels the very evolution of mankind. Unfortunately, today's grains are highly refined. We eat white rice, white bread, white pasta, and white flour—nutritionally empty calories. And of all the grains we do eat, Americans only eat a mere 1 percent of whole grains! Whole grains should be the very basis of your diet.

The real cure for blood sugar dysfunction of any kind is making better food choices and eating whole natural foods. Diet is everything! Read Chapter 5, "Diet, Diet, Diet." (See page 29). Eating fat, sugars, refined foods, and just plain too much food, is the basic cause of blood sugar problems. Eating whole, natural, high-fiber, low-fat, low-sugar foods is the cure. Supplements, hormones, and exercise are secondary to what you eat. You can cure diabetes and other conditions with diet alone, but that is difficult, takes longer, and is simply not necessary. Making the best food choices, taking proven supplements, maintaining hormone balance, and sensible fasting are all necessary for curing blood sugar dysfunction.

WHOLE GRAINS

While most Americans consume enough total grains on a daily basis, most of those grain servings are refined grains, and very few are whole grains. Whole grains such as wheat, rice, barley, corn, rye, oats, buckwheat, spelt, and millet should be the core of what you eat. This is very easy to do by eating such foods as whole grain pasta, whole grain breads, brown rice, oatmeal, steamed barley, whole grain breakfast cereals, polenta, and unrefined grain products of all kinds. Whole grains naturally provide a number of nutrients, such as dietary fiber, several B vitamins, and minerals. Refined grain products tend to be enriched with vitamins and iron after processing. They often provide less fiber than whole grains.

Be sure that the products you are buying contain whole grains. Read the labels carefully. Foods that are marketed as multi-grain, stone-ground, cracked wheat, bran, or 100-percent whole wheat are not necessarily a whole grain product. Check the ingredients list to identify a whole grain product. The first ingredient listed should be a whole grain. A diet rich in whole grains has been proven to contribute in lowering the risk of diabetes.

BEANS AND LEGUMES

Beans and legumes are very closely related to whole grains. Research has determined that beans and legumes are associated with a lower diabetes risk, as well as preventing heart disease and reducing cholesterol levels. Beans are high in protein, dietary fiber, minerals, lignans, and sterols, but low in fat and calories. A 4-ounce serving of pinto beans, for example, has a mere 117 calories and 1-percent fat calories. Be sure to include beans and legumes in your daily fare. Legumes are available dried or pre-cooked in cans, and they are an inexpensive food. When you learn to cook beans and use them in stews, soup, dips, and spreads, you'll come to enjoy them very much.

THE SCIENCE BEHIND THE FACTS

There are so many published human clinical trials on whole grains that we can't begin to mention them all. We'll stick to some of the largest. At the Famous Harvard School of Nutrition (*PLoS Medicine* v. 4, 2007), 161,737 women, aged thirty-seven to sixty-five, in the classic Nurses' Health Study were followed. Their dietary patterns were studied. The researchers concluded, "Whole grain intake is inversely associated with risk of type 2 diabetes. Findings from prospective cohort studies consistently support increasing whole grain consumption for the prevention of type 2 diabetes." You can just not debate the results from this many people studied over years. The more whole grains you eat, the less chance of getting diabetes or any other blood sugar disorder. More research from Harvard (*Annals of Internal Medicine* v. 136, 2002) was done with 42,504 men over a twelve-year period. This is 466,508 person years! A stunning review with twenty-four references was done at Harvard (*American Journal of Clinical Nutrition* v. 77, 2003), and they came to the very same basic conclusions.

At the University of Minnesota (*Proceedings of the Nutrition Society* v. 62, 2003), "Epidemiological Support For the Protection of Whole Grains Against Diabetes" was published. This impressive review was based on 160,000 men and women. "There is accumulating evidence to support the hypothesis that whole grain consumption is associated with a reduced risk of incident type 2 diabetes. It may also improve glucose control in diabetic individuals." They went on further to say, "Observations in non-diabetic individuals support an inverse relationship between whole grain consumption and fasting insulin levels." In other words, the more whole grains you eat, the more effective your insulin is metabolized. "Glucose control improved with diets rich in whole grain in feeding studies of subjects with type 2 diabetes." You cannot argue with the results of 160,000 people.

In a collective study between the USDA, Harvard, Tufts, and other institutions (*American Journal of Clinical Nutrition* v. 76, 2002), one of the famous Framingham series of studies was used to study whole-grain intake for the prevention of type 2 diabetes. "After adjustment for potential confounding factors, whole grain intake was inversely associated with body mass index, waist-to-hip ratio, total cholesterol, LDL cholesterol, and fasting insulin." They said further, "The inverse association between whole grain intake and fasting insulin was most striking among overweight participants." Their conclusion was, "Increased intake of whole grains may reduce disease risk by means of favorable effects on metabolic risk factors." The series of Framingham studies are the most prestigious ever done. In the very same journal, a similar study from Simmons College was published, which was entitled, "Whole Grain Intake and Risk of Type 2 Diabetes." As part of the Health Professionals Study, 51,529 men were followed for twelve years. This study is one of the most famous and best ever done. The dietary patterns of the men were examined in detail. Those who ate the most whole-grain foods had the least diabetes. Their conclusion was clear: "A diet high in whole grains is associated with a reduced risk of type 2 diabetes. Efforts should be made to replace refined grain with whole grain foods." Other similar published studies were done at Harvard with the very same results.

At the University of Minnesota, this same phenomenon was observed in 36,000 women for six years (*American Journal of Clinical Nutrition* v. 71, 2000). This was a first-rate study complete with forty-eight references. The more whole grains they ate, the less diabetes they suffered from. "These data support a protective role for whole grains, cereal fiber, and dietary magnesium in the development of diabetes in older women." The researchers found that, "Total grain, whole grain, total dietary fiber, and dietary magnesium intakes showed strong inverse correlations with incidence of diabetes." The more whole grains, the less diabetes.

Nathan Pritikin was a real natural health pioneer back in the 1980s. He published two articles (*Diabetes Care* v. 5, 1982 and v. 6, 1983) on diabetes, diet, and exercise. Diabetics on oral medication got off the drugs in just 26 days by simply eating a whole-grain based natural diet, and walking every day. In less than a month they were drug free! This is nothing less than amazing. The supplements we have today were not available at that time, nor were natural hormones like melatonin and DHEA. Eating better food and taking a daily walk got mostly all of them off medication in less than a month. Imagine the results Nathan could get today by adding proven supplements and natural hormones!

At Sun-Yatsen University in China (*Ying Xue-bao* v. 20, 1998) diabetics were fed legumes. This lowered their glucose levels as well as their C-peptide levels (a basic marker for heart disease). Tofu, by the way, is a heavily refined product that is lacking in nutrition, and should be used only occasionally.

CONCLUSION

Fiber is one of the important factors here. Whole grains and beans (legumes) have more soluble and insoluble fiber than any other food groups. Meat, poultry, eggs, and dairy products are completely lacking in fiber. There are many studies showing the importance of fiber, not only for blood sugar conditions, but for all major diseases. The best way to get fiber is by eating whole grains and beans every day. There are many studies to show that merely adding fiber to our diet improves glucose and insulin metabolism dramatically. Fiber supplements are obviously not the answer at all. Eating whole foods gives you plenty of fiber, especially whole grains, beans, vegetables, and fruits. Americans are generally very fiber-deficient from eating refined foods and too many animal products that are fiberless.

4. Fats and Oils

Fats and oils are often thought of as being unhealthy. However, we need a small amount of fat in our diet each day. Some types of fat are beneficial to your health and others are not. Saturated fats and trans fats, which are derived from vegetable oils, have been shown to lead to many health risks. Saturated fats raise your LDL (bad cholesterol) level and your total cholesterol level. Trans fats can also raise your LDL level and lower your HDL (good cholesterol) level. Unsaturated fats are derived from vegetables and plants. There are two types of unsaturated fatty acids, monounsaturated fats and polyunsaturated fats. These fats have been proven to lower your LDL cholesterol levels.

SATURATED FATS

Low-fat diets do not rule out fat entirely, but it is necessary to understand which fats should be avoided and which ones are healthy. Americans eat about 42 percent of their calories as saturated fats. You only need about 8 percent unsaturated vegetable oils, so this is more than 500 percent of what you need. These saturated fats are artery clogging fats. They are derived from animal products such as meat, dairy, and eggs. These saturated fats are the wrong kind of fats. It is a major reason we lead the world in heart disease, various cancers, diabetes, and other major illnesses.

We are addicted to animal fats. While various sugars are the main cause of diabetic-type conditions, saturated fats, as well as omega-6 fatty acids from vegetable oils, are another major factor. Fats and sugars work together synergistically to cause high insulin, high blood sugar, and increased insulin resistance. The combination is truly devastating.

VEGETABLE OILS

It is not just the saturated fats that cause problems, but also excess vegetable oils due to the omega-6 content. We eat far too many omega-6 fatty acids, and far too few omega-3s. This is why flax oil is recommended as a supplement. Flax is the best source of omega-3 fatty acids known. Yes, the Mediterranean diet is better than the Western European and American diets, but it is *not* the answer at all. Excessive intake of olive oil is just as harmful as any other vegetable oil. Vegetable oils are merely less harmful than animal fats. The point here is to eat a diet of less than 20-percent total fat. A 30-percent fat diet is not "low." There is also the problem of hydrogenated and partially hydrogenated trans fatty acids. These are made by forcing hydrogen gas into vegetable oil under extreme pressure with exotic catalysts. This "saturates" the molecule, and gives the oil longer shelf life. Hydrogenated fats are the worst possible choice, and you should avoid them. Read your labels. The published research in the last few years on the effect of dietary fats is far too voluminous to even attempt to cover. We certainly can mention a few of the largest reviews to prove this very clearly. The best evidence comes from an analysis of the free fatty acids (FFAs) in our plasma.

DIABETES AND HIGH-FAT DIETS

How do we know for a fact that high-fat diets cause diabetes and other blood sugar conditions? Epidemiologists have studied the patterns of health events, and consistently, epidemiological studies have shown that countries like China, Vietnam, Thailand, Korea, and Japan have far lower diabetes rates. However, migration studies have shown that when these people move to the United States and adopt the typical Western diet, they get as many, and usually *more*, blood sugar conditions than other Americans. Studies of what people eat also prove that the more fats—especially unhealthy fats—they consume, the higher the chance that they will get diabetes. When diabetics are given low-fat diets, they improve dramatically. Lastly, studies of the plasma free fatty acids (FFAs) in our blood give irrefutable proof that fats, especially saturated fats, cause blood sugar dysfunction.

OBESITY AND DIABETES

Obesity is not just an aesthetic issue, it is a health hazard. Obesity has been associated with diabetes and many other medical conditions such as heart disease, high blood pressure, cancer, and others. Sedentary lifestyles and convenient high-fat foods play a major role in obesity. We must discuss obesity in relation to fat intake. It is not food that makes you fat; it is fat that makes you fat. Dietary fat plays an important role in the development of obesity. When you reduce your fat intake it reduces that gap between your energy intake and your energy output. You simply cannot be overweight, or stay overweight, if you take dairy products, meat, poultry, and eggs out of your life. Overweight people always eat more fat and have much higher levels of free fatty acids in their blood. These fatty acids are mostly all those from animal foods, not those from vegetable sources. Being overweight places extra stress on your body in many ways. It may interfere with your body's ability to maintain safe blood glucose levels. It may cause your body to become insulin resistant, which can eventually cause you to develop diabetes.

THE SCIENCE BEHIND THE FACTS

The published research from just the last few years on the effect of dietary fats is far too voluminous to even attempt to cover. We certainly can mention a few of the largest reviews to prove this very clearly. The best evidence comes from an analysis of the free fatty acids (FFAs) in our plasma. At the University of Richmond (*Metabolism* v. 51, 2002), the effect of dietary fats on diabetes was reviewed in a study called, "The Role of Plasma Fatty Acid Composition in Patients with Type 2 Diabetes." This was a lengthy review with a full fifty-five references. Fourteen different fatty acids were analyzed from patients and controls. Overall, plasma saturated fatty acids (from animal fats) were 43-percent higher in diabetics. Specifically, saturated fatty acids like palmitic, oleic, and stearic were much higher in the diabetic patients. "Total saturated fatty acid (SFA) concentrations (350 versus 231 μmol/L) were significantly increased in the diabetic subjects." Please note, this is 350 μmol versus only 231 μmol. Vegetable oils did not play a part, but there was a deficiency of omega-3 fatty acids and an excess of omega-6. As usual, it was also found that diabetics had dramatically higher triglycerides, higher cholesterol, and lower HDL, as well as higher insulin and blood sugar. A detailed analysis of FFAs in human blood makes an inarguable case that animal fats in your diet cause blood sugar disorders.

This same phenomenon was demonstrated at the University of Minnesota (*American Journal of Clinical Nutrition* v. 78, 2003). In this study, 2,909 adults had the fatty acids in their blood measured. This is a better means to determine fat intake than mere dietary analysis. "Our findings suggest that the dietary fat profile, particularly that of saturated fat, may contribute to the etiology of diabetes." They further said, ". . . diabetes incidence was significantly and positively associated with the proportion of total saturated fatty acids in plasma." They specifically found high levels of saturated (animal) fatty acids such as palmitic, palmitoleic, and stearic in their blood. Again, we find animal products in the diet as the cause of diabetes.

The Women's Health Study (*Diabetes Care* v. 27, 2004) has been one of the largest and longest ongoing studies of female health, and involved more than 37,000 women over the age of forty-five. The amount of red meat they consumed was compared to their incidence of diabetes. "Our data indicate that higher consumption of total red meat, especially processed meats, may increase the risk of women developing type 2 diabetes." They also found that consumption of cholesterol and animal protein was significantly associated with high diabetes rates. These results were carefully adjusted to exclude other possible factors, like dietary fiber. Always remember that cholesterol is found only in animal foods, not plant foods.

We can further prove the relation of fat intake to blood sugar dysmetabolism with studies in which people change from high-fat to low-fat diets. This is especially true with regard to vegetable oils instead of animal fats. At the University of Otago in New Zealand (*British Journal of Nutrition* v. 83 Supp, 2000), a heavily referenced review of the literature in this area was published. "Lifestyle changes can reduce the progression of impaired glucose tolerance in type 2 diabetes. Insulin sensitivity is enhanced by a range of diet-related changes, including reduction of visceral adiposity, and a reduction in saturated fatty acids." Saturated fat intake causes diabetes—plain and simple.

Another powerful review, with forty-four references, from the University of Uppsala in Sweden (*British Journal of Nutrition* v. 83, 2000), found high levels of palmitic and palmitoleic fatty acids (from animal foods) in the blood serum of diabetics. FFAs were clearly related to both diabetes and obesity as well. "A high level of dietary fat is associated with impaired insulin sensitivity and risk of diabetes." Similar studies show significant relationships between serum lipid fatty acid composition, which mirrors the type, and amount of the fatty acids in the diet, and insulin sensitivity. You are just not going to have high levels of palmitic, palmoleic, and stearic acids in your blood when you eat whole grains, vegetables, fruits, and seafood as your basic sustenance, as these are basically not from saturated animal fats.

These results were verified by the Centre de Recherche in France (*Diabete & Metabolisme* v. 21, 1995) in a review with eighty-nine references. FFA levels were clearly and directly associated with diabetes and other blood sugar problems. Also, in a review with seventy-four references from Temple University in Arizona (*Diabetes* v. 46, 1997), FFA levels are elevated in obesity as well. At the University of Napoli in Italy, a twelve-page review with 131 references was done. In this study (*European Journal of Lipid Science* v. 103, 2001), they found plasma FFAs to be strongly correlated with high cholesterol, high blood pressure, high triglycerides, obesity, insulin resistance, coronary heart disease, and outright diabetes. That's pretty clear!

CONCLUSION

The literature is replete with studies such as these, and the scientific community is in good agreement that high-fat diets are one of the major causes of the growing epidemic of type 2 diabetes, and as well as other blood sugar problems. These studies validate that changes in diet and physical activity to achieve weight loss can prevent the development of type 2 diabetes in those who are at high-risk. Remember, a high-fat diet and excessive consumpton of saturated fat is associated with an increase in the risk of type 2 diabetes. Also, eating a "low-fat diet" means that no more than 20 percent of your food contains fat, and that most of the vegetable oils you consume contain unsaturated fat. This is very easy to do by simply taking animal products out of your diet and eating moderate (10 percent) amounts of seafood. In the next chapter, we will take a closer look at important dietary measures.

5. Diet, Diet, Diet

A wholesome, low-fat, natural foods diet, along with a healthy lifestyle and exercise, is the way to cure blood sugar conditions of all kinds. Diet is the very key to health more than any other factor. A diet based on whole grains, beans (all kinds), green and yellow vegetables, local fruits, soups, salads, and seafood (if you want) will allow you to live longer and have a much higher quality of life. Americans eat 42-percent fat calories, nearly all of which are from saturated animal fats. This is five times the amount of fat they need. They also eat twice the protein, half the fiber, and twice the amount of calories they need, plus 160 pounds of various sugars they don't need at all. We are overfed and undernourished. Traditional Japanese macrobiotics has a very limited selection of foods, and does not use supplements, natural hormones, rigorous exercise, or even fasting. The word "macrobiotics," simply means an overall (macro) view of life (bios). You eat the common foods you grew up with. There is really nothing exotic about it.

FATS

One of the basic causes of blood sugar dysmetabolism is a diet high in saturated animal fats. This is documented in the previous chapter. Americans eat over 500 percent of the fats they need, and nearly all of these are saturated animal fats instead of vegetable oils. You do not have to be a vegetarian to cure diabetes and similar illnesses, as 10 percent of your diet can consist of seafood. Ideally, you would eat no beef, pork, lamb, poultry, eggs, or dairy foods. Technically, diabetics could eat, say, three 4-ounce portions of lean meat every week and still cure themselves, but this would slow down your progress. The best way to cure yourself is to stop eating red meat, poultry, eggs, and all dairy products. This includes low-fat and lactose-reduced dairy products.

MILK PRODUCTS

Milk and milk products are the most allergic foods known. They contain lactose (milk sugar) and cancer-promoting casein. All adults of all races are lactose intolerant, since they no longer produce the enzyme lactase. Without lactase, you simply cannot digest lactose. It's a face that everyone over the age of three years old is allergic to dairy products. Nature provided cow milk for calves and goat milk for baby goats. Lactose-reduced milk is just not the answer here at all, nor is lactase tablets like Lactaid. Dairy cheese is low in lactose but extremely high in saturated animal fat, casein, and cholesterol. It is a very poor food choice. You can use soy, rice, almond, or oat milks instead of dairy milk. Very good meltable non-dairy cheeses are available at any grocery store. You can even buy soy cream cheese. Dairy yogurt has twice the amount of milk sugar, since powdered milk is added to thicken it. Soy yogurt and soy ice cream are readily available, but they contain quite a bit of sugar.

The studies proving that dairy products cause diabetes are numerous. At the Health Protection Branch in Canada (*American Journal of Clinical Nutrition* v. 51, 1995), the doctors said, "There is a significant positive correlation between consumption of milk protein and incidence of IDDM in data from various countries." They also found that babies who were naturally breast fed were protected from type 1 diabetes. At the A2 Corporation in New

Zealand (*Medical Hypotheses* v. 56, 2001), the researchers clearly found milk proteins related to diabetes, heart disease, and outright mortality. "Milk casein consumption also correlates strongly with type 1 diabetes incidence." At the University of Helsinki in Finland (*Experimental and Clinical Endocrinology & Diabetes* v. 105, 1997), the research showed clearly that milk consumption, both for mothers and children, is a major cause of type 1 diabetes. Again, at the University of Helsinki (*Diabetologia* v. 41, 1998), they found that the children who were most allergic to dairy products (based on blood antibodies) had the highest rates of diabetes. At the University of Tampere in Finland (*Diabetes* v. 49, 2000), they said, "In conclusion, our results provide support for the hypothesis that high consumption of cow's milk during childhood can be diabetogenic." At NIZO Research in the Netherlands (*Nahrung* v. 43, 1999), the same results were found. At the School of Medicine in Auckland, New Zealand (*Diabetologica* v. 42, 1999), it was clear that consumption of dairy products were strongly correlated with type 1 diabetes. The research is clear on this: Take dairy products completely out of your life. Milk is not good food.

BEANS

Beans are an excellent food and very similar to whole grains in their nutritional profile. There are many delicious varieties of beans available, especially in ethnic grocery stores. Beans, bean soups, and bean dips should be a central part of your daily fare. Get a good cookbook, and learn how to make more gourmet bean dishes. If you have problems with gas or bloating, this is not due to the beans, but rather to your weakened digestive system. Take Beano, or a generic version of alpha galactosidase, temporarily until your digestive system is stronger.

FISH AND SEAFOOD

Fish and seafood can be eaten by people who do not want to be vegetarians. If you look in your mouth, you will see we have canine teeth. The human diet can consist of about 10-percent food from animals, and the best choice is seafood. A few people are allergic to fish and seafood, however, and will not be able to eat them. Just limit seafood to about 10 percent of your diet. If you want to be a vegetarian or vegan, just don't eat seafood. There are no other animal products in the American macrobiotic diet.

PROTEIN

We eat twice the protein we need. This causes many health problems, including obesity, kidney disease, and liver disease. Many studies have proven that a high-protein diet raises uric acid, and causes kidney and liver problems. Anytime you hear an author advocating a high-protein diet, you will know they are clueless and uninformed. Whole grains, beans, and vegetables contain all the high-quality protein and fiber you need. There are many studies to prove this. At Nara Medical University (*Nara Igaku Zasshi* v. 46, 1995), the doctors concluded, "A protein-limited diet was useful for prevention of diabetic nephropathy in patients with early-stage diabetic nephropathy." At the University of Vermont (*American Journal of Physiology* v. 27, 1996), they found the same results. Decreased protein intake was found to improve symptoms of type 1 diabetes. Limit your protein intake.

VEGETABLES

Nearly all green and yellow vegetables are a good choice. However, you should avoid nightshades, most tropical vegetables, and those high in oxalic acid. Japanese macrobiotics does not include many green and yellow vegetables, ironically. Actually, frozen vegetables are very nutritious; only the texture is harmed by the freezing process. Canned vegetables should be avoided. Avoid the nightshade family. This includes potatoes, tomatoes, peppers, and eggplants. Nightshades contain large amounts of toxic solanine. Macrobiotics is about the only diet system to warn against these nightshade vegetables. Also avoid vegetables high in oxalic acid, such as spinach, Swiss chard, and others. Tropical vegetables, like taro, are meant for tropical people living in tropical climates. If you are of, say, African or Indian descent and living in southern Florida or Arizona, you certainly can eat such tropical foods. If you are of European descent, these foods are simply not meant for you.

You can eat a fresh green salad every day as long as you use a low-fat, non-dairy dressing. Traditional Japanese macrobiotics has a bias against fresh salads for some reason. In fact, they basically have a bias against all raw foods. The best time to eat salads is in summer time, since they are rather yin. You can still enjoy fresh salads all year round. People who advocate a 100-percent raw food diet are irrationally neurotic and cannot stay on these very long, as their health deteriorates so badly.

SUGARS

People with blood sugar dysmetabolism of any kind cannot eat fruit juice, dried fruits, or sweeteners of any type until they are well. Avoid sugar substitutes like stevia. If your pancreas has atrophied or has been removed, this means you have to remove sugar from your diet permanently. You might think fruits provide important nutrients and that your diet will be incomplete without them. This is not the case at all, since fruits are basically made up of simple sugars, fiber, and water with very few vitamins and minerals. You cannot use sweeteners, including honey, fructose, fruit juice, dried fruit, maple syrup, stevia, lo han, agave, molasses, rice syrup, corn syrup, or any others. Sugar is sugar is sugar, and honey is biologically no better than white sugar. Artificial sweeteners are the worst, and none of them are safe. The newest claim from sucralose, "Made from sugar, tastes like sugar," is just not true. They don't tell you this is a man-made halogenated (chlorine molecules are added), synthetic, chemical, unnatural analog that isn't safe for human or animal use. Kick the sugar habit, and take the concept of "desserts" out of your life. You don't need desserts or sweets. The concept of dessert basically does not exist in Asia.

Scientists in Japan concluded, "The main reason of recent increase of diabetic patients is ascribed to increased sucrose intake" (*Chiba Igaku Zasshi* v. 72, 1996). Folks, Americans eat more than 160 pounds of various sugars and sweeteners every year, which they don't need at all. The worst offender of all is high fructose corn syrup, since it is the cheapest to produce. At the Diabetes Research Centre in India (*Diabetologica* v. 44, 2001), it was shown that the urban (not rural) Indians have inordinately high sugar intake. This causes epidemic-like diabetes rates, even though they are largely vegetarian and eat a very low-fat diet. Eating sweets will raise your triglyceride levels dramatically, even without eating fats.

It will be difficult for some people to simply give up all sweets and fruits. You can go through a transition period where you eat no cakes, cookies, sodas, pies, candy, or any other high-sugar foods. For a few months, you can eat 10 percent fresh (not dried or juiced) local fruit. No tropical fruits, though, as these are meant for tropical people in tropical lands. This shows the link between genetics, climate, and the food you should eat. You can also get a macrobiotic dessert cookbook and make whole grain desserts, lightly sweetened with whole fruit only. You'll come to enjoy these, and the subtle sweetness will be enough for you. Remember, macrobiotic desserts are a temporary transition, and the sooner you take all fruit and sweeteners out of your diet, the faster you'll get well. Your body simply cannot handle simple sugars, regardless of how "natural" they are. Honey is still sugar. When you are fully cured, you can eat 10 percent local fresh (or frozen) fruit if you want.

SOUPS

You should enjoy a wide variety of natural soups. Eating soup will help you lose weight and stay slim. That's right; if you eat just two meals a day, and start with a delicious bowl of soup at each meal, you'll actually feel full and eat less food. Get some soup cookbooks, and learn to substitute healthier ingredients where meat, poultry, eggs, and dairy are called for. Traditional Japanese macrobiotics restrict you to only 5-percent soup daily, and almost always miso soup. There is just no reason for these kinds of unnecessary limitations. There is nothing magical or special about fermented soybeans. There are countless delicious soups you can make at home and freeze for future use.

THE SCIENCE BEHIND A HEALTHY DIET

What about real world published studies that 1) show the difference in cultural diets and rates of diabetes, and 2) diabetics who are given whole-food diets? At Pantox Laboratories in California (*Medical Hypotheses* v. 58, 2002), type 2 diabetics were given a natural vegan (no animal products) diet, along with daily walking. This study was backed up by a stunning 170 references. "The vegan diet/exercise strategy represents a safe, low-tech approach to managing diabetes that deserves far greater attention from medical researchers and practitioners." The patients got very quick, dramatic improvements and benefits, including basic changes in their very blood parameters. These patients were fed fresh local and tropical fruits. People with blood sugar problems should avoid fruit and fruit juice until they are cured. Both contain simple sugars such as sucrose and fructose.

A cross-sectional study was done at the famous Cambridge University (*British Journal of Nutrition* v. 83, 2000), and they concluded, "Healthy Balanced Diets as One of the Main Components of Disease Prevention." In this study, 802 people were given GTTs (glucose tolerance tests). It was clear that the ones who made better food choices had far less diabetes. The healthy people ate more vegetables, salads, fish, fruits, pasta, and rice. Those with poor GTT results generally ate more meat, dairy, eggs, and fried foods. In another study, 25,698 Seventh Day Adventist vegetarians were examined (*American Journal of Pub-*

lic Health v. 75, 1985). Adventists are known to have far lower rates of diabetes, cancer, heart disease, and other conditions as a whole. The people who did not eat eggs or dairy products were shown to be the healthiest. You can't argue with the results of almost 26,000 real men and women.

Doctors at UCLA gave almost 5,000 male and female diabetics a diet and exercise program (*Diabetes Care* v. 17, 1994) for just three weeks. Glucose levels fell dramatically. In just twenty-one days, 71 percent of the ones taking oral medication discontinued their drugs! That is over 70 percent in twenty-one days! Thirty-nine percent of those on insulin stopped injecting themselves! That is almost 40 percent getting off insulin in twenty-one days! They simply ate better foods and did some moderate exercise. Imagine what would happen if they did this for a whole year. These results are simply amazing!

We need to mention the Pima Indians again. Half the Pima Indians still live in Mexico and follow their ancient traditional diet and lifestyle. The others live in the southwestern United States, and have largely adopted the American lifestyle. Many studies have been done here because they are from the same genetic stock. This study (*Diabetes Care* v. 24, 2001), from the University of Pittsburg, looked at their diabetes rates. The Mexican Pimas ate more corn, beans, squash, melons, and desert plants. They actually ate more calories (they do more physical labor), but had lower glucose levels and far less diabetes. The American Pimas have a 50 percent diabetes rate, short life spans, and many other diseases from eating the usual high-fat, high-sugar, refined-food diet. American Pimas, given their native diet, decrease their disease rates immediately. This also shows that genetics is not the problem.

A fine review from the Helicon Foundation (*Medical Hypotheses* v. 54, 2000), with eighty-four references was titled, "Toward a Wholly Nutritional Therapy for Type 2 Diabetes." The authors suggest preventing and treating type 2 diabetes with only diet, supplements, and exercise rather than toxic, ineffective drugs.

They also point out that obesity, one of the most important causes of all, would be basically eradicated by such dietary means. We need more such progressive doctors using natural means to cure disease.

Another study from Harvard (*Annals of Internal Medicine* v. 136, 2002) was titled, "Dietary Patterns and Risk for Type 2 Diabetes in U.S. Men." Here, over 42,000 men aged forty to seventy-five were studied for diabetes, cancer, and heart disease for twelve years. It was clear that the ones who ate more whole grains, vegetables, fresh fruits, and fish lived the longest, and had the lowest illness rates. The ones who ate red meat, refined grains, dairy products, fried foods, and desserts had far higher disease rates and much shorter lives. Forty-two thousand real people prove the point conclusively.

The diet books in print are generally distressing, and there are very few authors who can give you the proper guidance. If you go to a bookstore or library, you will see many books claiming to tell you how to cure diabetes. Nearly all of them are not only useless, but may actually make you worse. You can always tell if the books are spurious if the author suggests eating dairy products, eggs, meat, poultry, sweeteners of any kind (including honey and stevia), tropical foods (like bananas and citrus), or nightshade vegetables (like potatoes and tomatoes). It is not considered "good form" in this business to mention these pseudo-authorities by name, so they won't be named individually. However, you will find a list of useful resources that I do recommend on page 119.

GLYCEMIC INDEX

The glycemic index must be mentioned. This theory is based on how much sugar in the foods we eat wind up going into your blood stream. The problem is that the glycemic index is extremely misleading. It labels good foods as high on the index, which is bad, and bad foods that are low on the index as good, which is extremely bad. What this means is that white bread, ice cream, and chocolate cake are good, and brown rice, oatmeal, and many fruits are bad. The fact is, if whole grains raised blood sugar, all Asian countries would have the highest rates of diabetes in the world. Instead, they consume the most grains and have the lowest rates of diabetes.

The problem is that this theory has begun to enter the mainstream through medical journals and advertising. The underlying idea is simple. Eat foods with a low-glycemic index, such as red meat, poultry, eggs, and dairy foods, and you can be lean and healthy. This is far from the truth. Do not be misled. Let common sense and science based on traditional diets guide you to a better way to eat.

CALORIE INTAKE

Calorie restriction is an important part of curing blood sugar conditions. Americans eat twice the amount of the calories they need. We eat three meals a day when we only need two. Be sure to eat two meals a day instead of three. You need to eat only twice a day, and soon this will become perfectly normal for you. Breakfast is not, "the most important meal of the day." The less calories you eat, the longer you live. Men can thrive on about 1,800 calories a day, and women on about 1,200 calories. Roy Walford is the only one who wrote extensively on this subject. Please read his books, *The 120 Year Diet* and *Maximum Lifespan*. Eat as little as possible, and keep your caloric intake down by eating low fat foods. It isn't food that makes you fat; it is fat that makes you fat. You don't need to walk around hungry, nor can you. Willpower is an illusion. You can eat all you want, and still take in fewer calories by simply making better food choices. You can eat all you want, never be hungry, and still stay slim if you just eat whole, natural foods. The answer is eating lower-fat foods and not less food. Please take a good look at the calorie density chart in Chapter 13 on obesity (page 105), to convince yourself of this. You can literally eat all you want, if you just make better food choices. Americans eat twice the amount of the calories they need.

It would literally take eighty years to study humans for the total benefits of calorie restriction, but we have 1) shorter-term human studies, and 2) full-term animal studies. Calorie restriction is the most effective way to extend lifespan and quality of life. At Heinrich-Heine University in Germany, a heavily referenced review was published (*Weiner Klinische Wochen* v. 106, 1994). Real people greatly improved their insulin sensitivity and lost weight by eating lower calorie foods. At the Franco-Czech Laboratory (*Journal of Clinical Endocrinology & Metabolism* v. 89, 2002), obese women improved their insulin resistance and lost weight simply by eating lower calorie foods. At Alexandra Hospital (*International Journal of Obesity* v. 27, 2003), obese diabetic men were given lower calorie foods for twelve weeks. They lost weight, lost body fat, lowered their cholesterol, and improved glycemic control with no other intervention. At Nagasaki University (*International Congress Series* v.1209, 2000), diabetic women were fed a low-calorie, low-fat diet based on rice and vegetables. Their glycemic status improved, and their glucose levels fell significantly.

FASTING

Fasting is always a part of any serious natural health program. With most blood sugar disorders it can be difficult to fast on water even for twenty-four hours, from dinner to dinner. If you want to know more, the recommended books on fasting are listed in *Zen Macrobiotics for Americans*. When you are cured, it is important you fast one day a week on water, from dinner to dinner. This gives your body fifty-two times every year to rest, recuperate, and heal. Once you see the great benefits, you'll probably choose to do longer fasts. If you can go twenty-four hours on water only, without problems, then you should do this for one day every week, from dinner to dinner.

CONCLUSION

Billions of dollars are wasted every year treating the *symptoms* of obesity, because we refuse to look at the *cause* of this overweight epidemic. Americans basically eat high-fat, low-bulk, low-fiber, calorically dense, highly refined, high-sugar foods. We are overfed and undernourished. If you eat a high-fat diet, you will have high body fat. Vegetable oils are just as fattening as animal fats and have the same amount of calories. You are what you eat, and the more fat you eat, the fatter you will be. Maintaining a low-fat, high-fiber, and low-sugar diet will decrease your chances of suffering from a blood sugar condition.

6. Effective Supplements

It cannot be emphasized enough: What you eat is the real cure for blood sugar and insulin dysmetabolism. Your daily food is basically what will cure you. Whole natural foods cure disease. Proven supplements and natural hormones are very powerful, but secondary to diet. Supplements are only one of the Seven Steps to Natural Health (see page 117). People are understandably confused about which supplements work, and which are merely advertising promotions. This confusion can be explained in one word—*advertising*. To know which supplements honestly have value, we merely need to look at the published scientific literature, rather than the very well-written advertisements that inundate us. Science, not skillful ad writers, tells us which supplements really benefit us.

TAKING SUPPLEMENTS

First, we need to understand the difference between "endogenous" supplements and "exogenous" ones. *Endogenous supplements* exist in our bodies and in the common foods we eat. This would include all vitamins, all minerals, all basic hormones, most amino acids, and such supplements as CoQ_{10}, beta-sitosterol, lipoic acid, DIM, PS, and beta glucan. You can, and should, take the appropriate and needed endogenous supplements for the rest of your life for your general health. This is especially true if you are over forty years of age. People under forty need only acidophilus, FOS, beta glucan, vitamin D, vitamin E, flax oil, minerals, and vitamins.

Acetyl-L-Carnitine (ALC)

Acetyl-L-carnitine (ALC) is the preferred form of L-carnitine, as it is more bioavailable and passes into the brain more easily. There are a number of studies on both forms, but you will get all the benefits of plain L-carnitine by taking the acetyl deriva-tive ALC. At the Instituto di Medicina in Italy (*Metabolism* v. 49, 2000), type 2 diabetics were given ALC. This effectively increased their glucose disposal and utilization. They conclud-ed this was an important therapy. ALC is an important supple-ment for anyone over forty for brain function, memory, and clarity of thought.

DOSAGE: An appropriate dose is 500 mg a day.

Acidophilus

Acidophilus keeps the good bacteria in our intestines alive. Find a good refrigerated brand and keep it refrigerated. This will help strengthen your digestion.

DOSAGE: Take 6 billion units (with 8 strains) once or twice daily, and use FOS (see page 45) and L-glutamine (see page 46) with it.

Beta Carotene

Beta carotene has been shown to be deficient in most diabetics, but not vitamin A. (Beta carotene is the direct precursor to vitamin A.) Beta carotene is one of the most powerful anti-oxidants in our diet. Some studies, such as the one done at Jikei University in Japan, show high serum vitamin A levels, but low levels of beta carotene. This is a very effective anti-oxidant, and should definitely be a part of your program. The

Third National Health and Nutrition Examination Survey (*Diabetes* v. 52, 2003) showed low levels of carotenoids (except lycopene) generally in diabetics.

DOSAGE: You only need 10,000 IU here, although you can take 25,000 for the first year if you want to.

Beta Glucan

Beta glucan is a very important supplement to take for all forms of sugar dysmetabolism. Beta glucan is the most powerful immune enhancer known to science, including interferon-alpha. It doesn't matter whether you use oat or yeast glucan, as all are one-third true glucans. The mushroom glucan is simply too expensive. A good number of human studies have shown the benefits of beta glucan for all blood sugar issues. Beta glucan also has powerful cholesterol- and triglyceride-lowering activity, which, of course, is of great concern in blood sugar dysmetabolism. This is a very important supplement that you must add to your regimen, and even healthy children and people under forty should routinely take this. Eat just a little oatmeal and barley regularly, and you won't need to take a supplement.

DOSAGE: The usual dosage is 200 mg, but you should take 400 mg for the first year to improve glycemic control.

Beta-Sitosterol

Beta-sitosterol is found in every vegetable you eat, but there just isn't enough in our daily food. It is estimated the average American eats about 300 mg daily, while vegetarians eat twice that amount. Vegetarians have far less blood sugar problems. Beta-sitosterol is the most effective natural remedy known for both prostate problems and high blood fats (cholesterol and triglycerides). At the Gerontology Clinic (*Vnitrni Lekarstvi* v. 50, 2004), blood levels of these plant sterols were shown to be very important in diabetic patients. "In diabetics the level of disease compensation correlated negatively with plant sterol values." All this is strongly related to cholesterol and triglyceride dysmetabolism.

DOSAGE: Take 300 mg a day of mixed sterols (mixed sterols is the only form available). You should take 600 mg a day for the first year, and then just 300 mg.

CoQ$_{10}$

CoQ$_{10}$ is a basic supplement. Some unscrupulous companies offer smaller amounts of CoQ$_{10}$ with "special delivery systems." These are all but worthless; 100 mg is what you need. Some "experts" recommend 300 to 400 mg a day, but this is a waste of money and not necessary at all. Real Japanese bioengineered CoQ$_{10}$ can be found (60 X 100 mg) for under $20. Studies around the world have shown the importance of this for diabetes. For example, at Moradabad Hospital in India (*Antioxidants in Human Health and Disease* 1999), a review with fifty-nine references on the benefits of CoQ$_{10}$ for diabetes and CHD was published. CoQ$_{10}$ is a powerful and basic supplement.

DOSAGE: You must take 100 mg of real Japanese ubiquinone a day. Do not take ubiquinol! Ubiquinol is unstable and has no shelf life.

Diindolylmethane (DIM)

Diindolylmethane (DIM) is a fine supplement, and better than I3C (indole-3-carbinol) for improving estrogen metabolism. If you test your free estradiol and estrone levels, and find them to be in the low normal (the ideal) range, you won't need to take this. Men over the age of fifty generally have higher estradiol and estrone levels than their postmenopausal wives! Excess estrogen in men or women is harmful, and low normal levels are best. American and European women rarely have insufficient estrogen levels due to their high-fat, low-fiber, nutrient-deficient diets, as well as obesity, lack of exercise, and other factors. Asian women who have low estradiol and estrone (but not estriol) levels have less heart disease, osteoporosis, and menopausal problems. The idea that American women generally are somehow "estrogen-deficient" after menopause is silly.

DOSAGE: Take 200 mg of DIM daily. All "special delivery systems" are just expensive advertising promotions. DIM is oil-soluble, so just take it with your food or with flax oil.

Flaxseed Oil

Flaxseed oil is the best source of omega-3 fatty acids and better than fish oil for a lot of reasons. All the studies on fish oil would be even more effective with flax oil. We eat far too many omega-6 fatty acids and far too few omega-3s. The research is overwhelming on the benefits of omega-3 supplementation for health blood sugar metabolism, as well as CHD health and blood lipids. At North Dakota University (*Nutrition Journal* v. 44, 2011), "Flaxseed Supplementation Improved Insulin Resistance in Obese Glucose Intolerant People" was published. The results were no less than dramatic. There are many such studies using real flax seed to help cure diabetes and other blood sugar issues. The research here is too much to continue with. This is a definite!

DOSAGE: Regardless of your age, take a 1,000 mg flax oil capsule every day, or one-half teaspoon of bulk flax oil. Buy and keep this refrigerated. Do not buy unrefrigerated flax oil, as it easily oxidizes.

Fructooligosaccarides (FOS)

Fructooligosaccarides (FOS) are indigestible sugars that feed the good bacteria in our intestines, but not the "bad" bacteria. This will not help blood sugar dysmetabolism directly, but will help keep your intestines healthy to better digest your food which helps normalize glucose metabolism. This supplement keeps our digestive system strong and healthy.

DOSAGE: Taking 750 mg once or twice a day works very well with acidophilus (see page 42) and L-glutamine (see page 46).

Glucosamine

Glucosamine will not specifically help your blood sugar condition, but it is an important supplement for anyone over the age of forty. Literally 95 percent of Americans over the age of sixty-five suffer from arthritis and joint inflammation. Do not take chondroitin, as it is not absorbed by our intestines and is therefore useless. Glucosamine cannot work alone; you must take a complete supply of minerals, flax oil, and vitamin D for it to be effective.

DOSAGE: Take 500 to 1,000 mg a day. It is a proven supplement for bone and joint health.

L-Glutamine

L-glutamine is an amino acid proven to promote good intestinal health. This will also spike or temporarily raise your growth hormone levels. While L-glutamine has shown no specific value for blood sugar problems, always remember we are treating the whole body, not just our glucose metabolism. Regardless of our age, our digestive systems are generally in terrible shape from our poor diets. Taking L-glutamine, with a good brand of acidophilus and FOS (see pages 42 and 45), will help us digest our food well. Strong digestion is an important part of maintaining normal blood sugar and insulin levels.

DOSAGE: You should take 1 g (two x 500 mg) in the morning and 1 g in the evening. You can also take 1 tablespoon (tbsp) of inexpensive bulk glutamine powder every day for even better results.

Glutathione

Glutathione is our other basic antioxidant enzyme. You can take oral glutathione, but it is not as effective as NAC. NAC is *N-acetyl cysteine*, which is a much more effective way to raise your glutathione levels than glutathione itself. The other varied benefits of NAC have been well documented in the last ten years. In diabetic conditions, glutathione has been shown to be of great importance because it is so basic to our antioxidant process. This is a vital supplement for blood sugar conditions, and much research has been done here.

DOSAGE: Take 600 mg of NAC a day.

Lipoic Acid

Lipoic acid has so much research on it, therefore I have provided a separate chapter devoted to the many international published studies on its benefits. See Chapter 8, "Alpha Lipoic Acid," on page 63.

Phospharidyl Serine (PS)

Phosphatidyl serine (PS) is a relative of lecithin or phosphatidyl choline. Only in the last few years has inexpensive PS become available to the public, and human research has verified its value. This is not going to help glycemic control per se, but you are treating your total health, not just glucose metabolism. Pregnenolone and acetyl-L-carnitine work very well with PS.

DOSAGE: Take 100 mg a day if you are over the age of forty to support good brain function. You can also benefit from taking a 1,200 mg softgel of lecithin for both better brain metabolism and lower cholesterol and triglyceride levels.

Soy Isoflavones

Soy isoflavones have been part of the diets of certain populations for centuries. It is unrealistic to think we are going to get a sufficient intake of these valuable isoflavones by eating a variety of soy products. Tofu is the white bread of soybeans, highly refined, and lacking in nutrition. Westerners rarely eat any amount of soy products such as miso, seitan, soy flour, tempeh, or other traditional Asian foods. Soy sauce is merely a condiment. There is an overwhelming amount of published research on the benefits of soy supplementation. Anyone who tells you soy is "bad" for you is mentally deficient. The dairy and meat industries are very upset by the popularity of soy products, especially soy milks. For centuries, billions of Asians have proven the value of soy isoflavone intake. Okinawans eat more soy than anyone and live the longest of all.

DOSAGE: Can be taken in 40 mg doses of combined genistein and daidzein.

Superoxide Dismutase (SOD)

Superoxide dismutase (SOD) is one of our two main antioxidant enzymes. Unfortunately, oral SOD pills don't work, nasal sprays are illegal, sublingual SOD isn't available, and the use of DMSO transdermal solutions is prohibited. Oral SOD tablets are worthless. Doctors don't know how to inject this, and it wouldn't be practical anyway. Nevertheless, SOD is very important to blood sugar problems because of the antioxidant stress. The University of Tiemcen in Algeria found low SOD blood levels in type 2 (but not in type 1) diabetics. Hyogo University, in Japan, found low SOD in type 1. By eating well, exercising, balancing your basic hormones, not taking prescription drugs, and avoiding negative habits (such as coffee, alcohol, cigarettes, recreational drugs), you will have higher SOD levels.

DOSAGE: We can keep our SOD levels elevated with diet, supplements, exercise, lifestyle, and generally supporting our antioxidant defense system.

VITAMINS

Vitamins, as well as *minerals,* are basic. There are only thirteen vitamins. Never take megadoses of any vitamin (or other supplement), as these overdoses unbalance our metabolism. Minerals are so important they are covered in a separate chapter. See Chapter 9, "The Minerals You Need" on page 69.

Vitamin B$_{12}$

Regular *Vitamin B$_{12}$* is not orally absorbed, so methycobalamin is most effective. You should find one with 1mg of methycobalamin, instead of a regular B$_{12}$ vitamin.

DOSAGE: Choose a supplement with 1 mg of methylcobalamin as the preferred form of B$_{12}$.

Vitamin C

Vitamin C is a very overrated and misunderstood vitamin. Megadoses of this will acidify your normally alkaline blood. Making the blood pH acidic will cause your entire system to be sickly. Megadoses of *anything*—including oxygen, sun, fun, food, sex, or whatever else—are harmful! Understand this simple fact. Vitamin C is only basically found in any quantity in tropical fruits, such as citrus. These are meant for tropical people in hot climates. You find very little vitamin C in temperate climate fruits and vegetables. Linus Pauling was wrong! Short-term studies of megadoses of vitamin C may show limited benefits, but never in the long term.

DOSAGE: Diabetics use up excessive vitamin C due to the increased need for all antioxidants. Therefore, you should take 250 mg until you are well. The RDA is only 60 mg. Again, do not take more than 250 mg, as this is four times the RDA.

Vitamin D

Vitamin D is not a vitamin at all, but rather a hormone. It does not occur in our food, except very small amounts in a few animal foods such as eggs. This is the most important "vitamin" of all for blood sugar problems. In the summer, if you get regular exposure to the sun, you can just take the 400 IU in your vitamin supplement. Most Americans are clearly deficient in "vitamin" D, as most of us do not get out in the sun regularly, especially in winter months. Science has proven that low vitamin D levels are an epidemic, correlated with endless illnesses, and clearly related to all-cause mortality and length of life. The international research is very strong here.

DOSAGE: Your daily vitamin supplement should have 400 IU, but you should take another 400 to 800 IU for many reasons. You should be getting a total of 800 to 1,200 IU of vitamin D per day, unless you are out in the sun regularly.

Vitamin E

Vitamin E is the second most important vitamin for blood sugar problems. Vitamin E is also very deficient in our diets because we eat a mere 1 percent whole grains (the main source). Always use the natural mixed tocopherols for a few dollars more, and not the inexpensive single tocopherol (d-alpha). The international published research on this is simply overwhelming. Vitamin E is one of the most powerful of all the natural antioxidants and must be a part of your healing program. This is very good for your heart and arteries. Hunan Medical University gave vitamin E to type 2 diabetics, which had dramatic benefits in only thirty days. The University of Chieti, in Italy, showed significant benefits in only fourteen days in type 2 diabetics. Vitamin E supplementation should be standard practice. The research here is obviously overwhelming and can't possibly all be quoted. People of all ages should use vitamin E, since we get so little in our diets.

DOSAGE: You should only use 200 IU a day (or 400 IU every other day). Do not exceed this, since the RDA is only 30 IU.

AN OVERVIEW OF IMPORTANT DAILY SUPPLEMENTS

The table below lists the most important supplements you should take on a permanent basis in order to help lower your cholesterol and to maintain good health in general. Next to the name of each supplement, you'll find the optimal daily intake, which is not necessarily the same as the Reference Daily Intake

(RDI) established by the Food and Drug Administration (FDA). Note, for example, that the RDI for vitamin E is only 30 IU, but the *optimal* daily intake is 200 IU.

TABLE 6.1. PERMANENT DAILY SUPPLEMENTS		
SUPPLEMENTS	OPTIMAL DAILY INTAKE	CONSIDERATIONS
VITAMINS		
Biotin	300 mcg	
Folate (Folic Acid)	400 mcg	
Pantothenic Acid	10 mg	
Vitamin B_1 (Thiamine)	1.5 mg	
Vitamin B_2 (Riboflavin)	1.75 mg	
Vitamin B_3 (Niacin)	20 mg	
Vitamin B_6	2 mg	
Vitamin B_{12}	2 mg	
Vitamin C	60 mg	Do not take more than 250 mg per day.
Vitamin D	800 IU	If you are sick or elderly, take up to 1,200 IU per day.
Vitamin E	200 IU of mixed natural tocopherols	Or take 400 IU every other day.
Vitamin K	80 mcg	
MINERALS		
Boron	3 mg	
Calcium	250 mg	Some suggest taking 1,000 mg of calcium per day, but only dairy intake will give you this much calcium, and it is better to avoid eating dairy.
Cesium	100 mcg	
Chromium	120 mcg	
Cobalt	100 mcg	

Supplements	Optimal Daily Intake	Considerations
Copper	2 mg	
Gallium	100 mcg	
Germanium	100 mcg	
Iodine	150 mcg	
Iron	10 mg for men, 18 mg for women	
Magnesium	400 mg	
Manganese	2 mg	
Molybdenum	75 mcg	
Nickel	100 mcg	
Selenium	70 mcg	
Silicon	10 mg	
Strontium	1 mg	
Tin	100 mcg	
Vanadium	1 mg	
Zinc	15 mg	
OTHER NUTRIENTS		
Acidophilus	6 billion live multi-strain organism capsules	Buy and keep refrigerated. Take once or twice daily.
Acetyl-L-Carnitine	500 to 1,000 mg	
Beta Carotene	10,000 IU	
Beta Glucan	200 mg or more	
Beta-Sitosterol	300 to 600 mg	
Coenzyme Q_{10} (CoQ_{10})	100 mg	If you are ill, take 200 mg daily for one year. Take with food or flax oil, as coenzyme Q_{10} is oil-soluble.
Diindolylmethane (DIM)	200 mg	Take with food or flax oil, as DIM is oil-soluble.

SUPPLEMENTS	OPTIMAL DAILY INTAKE	CONSIDERATIONS
Flaxseed Oil	1,000 to 2,000 mg	Buy and keep refrigerated. Take once or twice daily.
Fructooligosac-charides (FOS)	750 to 1,500 mg	
Glucosamine	500 to 1,000 mg	
L-glutamine	2,000 mg	Take two 500 mg tablets in the AM and two in the PM.
Lipoic Acid	400 mg	
N-acetyl Cysteine (Glutathione)	600 mg	
Phosphatidylserine (PS)	100 mg	
Quercetin	100 mg	
Soy Isoflavones	40 mg of daidzein and genistein	If you drink soy milk regularly, you probably don't need this.

CONCLUSION

A complete program of natural supplements is vital for healing, but it will never compensate for poor diet, lack of exercise, and other basic factors. Too often our diets lack the proper nutrients. Yet, with so many different nutrients available on the market, it is difficult to determine which ones you actually need. By understanding the role the nutrients discussed in this chapter play in maintaining good health, along with a naturally healthy diet and lifestyle, you can better understand how they can work effectively toward preventing and curing diabetes, as well as maintaining general good health. However, as you will see in the following chapters, there are other important elements to consider when creating a comprehensive program for yourself.

7. Temporary Supplements

As discussed in the previous chapter, endogenous supplements exist naturally in our bodies and in our daily food. These include all the ones mentioned in the previous chapter. On the other hand, exogenous supplements do not exist naturally in our bodies or our daily food. Before taking any of these supplements, it is important to understand what they are, how much to take, and how often. In this chapter, we will look at the most important of these supplements.

TAKING SUPPLEMENTS

Exogenous supplements are generally extracted from plants and herbs. This would include such items as ginseng, echinacea, milk thistle, golden seal, green tea, curcumin, guggul, ellagic acid, and aloe vera. It is important to point out that even if these supplements are appropriate for you, the effect will only last for about six months to a year and then cease. To continue taking them would be a waste of time and money, and could even be counterproductive. In fact, many people are allergic to some of these exogenous products. Therefore, all of these supplements should be taken for only up to twelve months, and then discontinued. Exogenous supplements should be temporary.

Aloe Vera

Aloe vera is a classic healing herb that helps our digestive system and our liver, among other benefits.

DOSAGE: Taking 2 x 100 mg capsules of a 200 to 1 extract is easier than trying to drink the equivalent of 40 g of fresh gel. Aloe gel is 99.5 percent water. Take for just six to twelve months, as it is exogenous.

L-arginine

L-arginine is an overrated and promoted amino acid with little scientific evidence behind it. There are a few possible studies, however, for blood sugar conditions. At the University of Vienna, L-arginine was found to inhibit lipid peroxidation in human diabetics. At the Medical College of Wisconsin, diabetic rats benefited from L-arginine in their water. At Cumhuriyet University in Turkey, rabbits had lowered blood glucose levels after ingesting oral L-arginine. Arginine is commonly promoted without clinical backing. This is an optional supplement, as its benefits are not clinically well proven at all.

DOSAGE: You can use 3 grams (6 x 500 mg) daily for one year.

Curcumin

Curcumin is a well-studied and time-proven antioxidant from the turmeric root. It is a natural supplement that is used to help improve digestive problems and blood glucose levels associated with diabetes. You need all the antioxidants you can get when treating insulin resistance.

DOSAGE: Take in 500 mg amounts daily for six months to a year. It is a powerful and proven natural antioxidant.

Ellagic Acid

Ellagic acid has no proof of efficacy for blood sugar disorders per se, but has shown very powerful anticancer and other effects.

DOSAGE: Take 100 mg a day for six months to a year to help your immunity in general.

Ginseng

Asian or American *ginseng* can be used temporarily, but not in hot weather or in tropical climates because of its extreme yang (warm) nature.

DOSAGE: Find a reliable brand, and take one or two capsules a day during the coolest six months of the year (October through March in the Northern Hemisphere).

Green Tea

Green tea extract is very worthwhile. Green tea is simply regular old tea (*Thea sinensis*) that is not fermented. There is a lot of good research on green tea polyphenols, but all of it is short-term only. It must have the caffeine removed to be safe or it is rather worrisome. This must be decaffeinated! It is unlikely you will drink two cups of decaf green tea every day, so the capsules are much more practical.

DOSAGE: Just take two capsules daily.

Milk Thistle

Milk thistle is the most effective herb for liver health. Milk thistle is the most researched herb for liver health, but it is exogenous and will not help you after a year. There are many human studies on the active ingredient silymarin.

DOSAGE: Take two capsules of a good extract every day for one year. It will work with the TMG (see page 59) to strengthen your liver.

Polysaccharide Plant Gums

Polysaccharide plant gums such as *glucomannan, guar gum, pectin* (citrus or apple), and *sodium alginate* (from seaweed) are very valuable, inexpensive, and safe temporary supplements. These plant gums have been shown to have value in lowering cholesterol, normalizing blood sugar, removing toxic metals, and other benefical functions. The added rewards of lowering cholesterol and triglycerides will be an important factor in your healing. Some people have lost weight using these, since the gums swell up dramatically with water and fill the stomach. This gives you a feeling of having eaten when you haven't. The science here is very strong. "Modified" citrus pectin is expensive and has no benefits at all. Buy regular inexpensive fruit pectins. At the 7th Annual Gums and Stabilizers Conference in England, researchers reviewed the benefits of these gums and found "improved glycemic control and a reduction in plasma cholesterol," which, of course, are precursors to diabetes. At the University of Helsinki, a review with fifty-nine references was published showing guar gum therapy had favorable long-term effects on glycemic control and lipid levels in NIDDM subjects. At St. Marianna University in Japan (*Eiyogaku Zasshi* v. 56, 1998), galactomannan (from fenugreek) was found to benefit by feeding 5 g a day to type 2 diabetics. At the Institute of Investigations in Cuba, guar, pectin, and glucomannan were all shown to help remove toxic heavy metals from the blood, improve digestion generally, and lessen the effects of diabetes.

DOSAGE: Take at least 3 g a day (6 x 500 mg capsules) to get real benefits. Choose the one you prefer or the one that is least expensive, or try each of the four above for three-month periods successively.

Quercetin

Quercetin is technically an endogenous antioxidant, although it is basically found only in apples and onions. Only one study was found where diabetic animals improved with quercetin supplementation. There is good science on the antioxidant benefits of quercetin.

DOSAGE: You can take 100 mg daily for one year.

Taurine

Taurine finally has good human science behind it for diabetes. Numerous animal studies showed great promise here, and now real people verify this. This inexpensive amino acid also has much value for coronary heart conditions generally, and helps lower blood fats and blood pressure. Studies at Beijing Hospital in China, Cardiology Research Center in Moscow, Bengbu Medical College in China, and Research University in Italy all showed improvement in glucose levels, insulin sensitivity, blood parameters, and other benefits in patients with both type 1 and 2 diabetes. Studies at the University of Messina and diabetes unit in Italy showed diabetics had low blood plasma and platelet taurine levels. In 2004, an extensive review of the literature with 114 references from the University of Sassari in Italy showed that taurine supplementation is valuable in treating diabetes and insulin resistance. Take for no more than one year.

DOSAGE: Take 500 mg of taurine daily for one year.

TMG

TMG (betaine), or trimethylglycine, is the most powerful liver rejuvenator known. The liver is the largest internal organ and vital to blood sugar metabolism. Our livers supply glycogen (blood sugar). Liver problems, especially such conditions as fatty liver, are central to blood sugar problems. TMG is a very important addition to your healing program. The human studies are excellent. To cure diabetes, you must have a strong healthy liver.

DOSAGE: Taking 3 g a day (6 X 500 mg capsules) for six months to a year will do wonders to cleanse and strengthen your liver. While TMG is endogenous, there is just no reason to use this much for more than a year. You can take 1 g (2 X 500 mg) as a permanent supplement after this.

Vitamin C

Vitamin C was covered in the previous chapter. It must be emphasized that megadoses weaken your immunity in the long run. It is *not* a dietary deficiency of vitamin C here at all, but rather the fact that the body is using up all the vitamin C and other antioxidants it can get to balance the free radicals.

DOSAGE: You should only take 250 mg for a year, and then the 60 mg in your vitamin supplement is enough as a permanent one. Never overdose on this!

SUPPLEMENTS TO AVOID

Nopal cactus has been promoted for normalizing blood sugar levels, but where is the evidence? There are no human or animal studies published in any of the international medical journals. There is just no reason to use something unproven like this when you have so many proven supplements to use. Bitter melon (*Momordica*) has also been promoted for blood sugar problems, but again, where is the evidence? Banaba leaf has corosolic acid in it and has been promoted for blood sugar problems. The published evidence is just not convincing so far. Fenugreek herb (containing galactomannan fiber) has been commercially promoted for diabetes, but the science is lacking here, too. In addition, conjugated linoleic acid (CLA) has been promoted for weight loss as well as diabetes, but again, the evidence just is not there.

The herb most promoted for normalizing blood sugar is *Gymnema sylvestre*. There are just no valid human studies here. Remember that exogenous supplements will not work for some people and will be biologically incompatible (allergenic) in others. If you feel any of these temporary supplements are not compatible with your individual biochemistry, then drop them. Some people will get mild side effects from exogenous supplements like these.

CONCLUSION

Always remember that a continuous effort to make better food choices is the most important thing we can do for our health. Natural health is about diet and lifestyle. Supplements are important, but they are secondary to diet. You receive far more health benefits with proper diet and both endogenous and exogenous supplements than with diet alone. In the following chapters we will be discussing the other nutrients that are vital in preventing and curing diabetes naturally.

8. Alpha Lipoic Acid

Alpha lipoic acid, or lipoic acid, levels in our bodies fall as we age, and unfortunately, this supplement is not found in our food. There are a lot of excellent scientific studies that suggest that lipoic acid is good for brain metabolism, coronary heart health, and blood sugar metabolism. Insulin resistance and diabetes are epidemics in Western society. Lipoic acid (thioctic acid), or "LA," is a natural antioxidant in our bodies. This is the most important single supplement you can take for diabetes and blood sugar disorders. Your blood sugar should be 85 mg/dL or less, and lipoic acid can help you achieve healthy blood sugar levels. It does not exist in the free form in our bodies, but rather as dihydrolipoic acid (DHLA). You are not going to get any from your diet. Do not think this is a magic supplement that can work alone. Diet and exercise is the basic cure for blood sugar dysmetabolism, while supplements and hormones play a secondary role. The research on lipoic acid is so overwhelming that we are going to devote a separate chapter to it.

WHAT IS LIPOIC ACID?

Lipoic acid (LA) is a disulfide (two sulfur atoms) that is converted in the body to dihydrolipoic acid, or DHLA. The lipoic acid of commerce, and the one used in nearly all the studies, is equally composed of two mirror image (*racemic*) isomers, R-isomer and S- isomer. Almost every one of the published studies uses the regular racemic natural R/S form. You will see Internet advertisements claiming that only the very expensive R-isomer has biological value, while the S-isomer is somehow ineffective. R-only lipoic acid is a promotion for money with no science behind it! Do not be taken in by such unfounded unscientific promotions. Clinical studies using these R- and S-forms separately found that they equally convert to DHLA (*General Pharmacology* v. 29, 1997). Just use regular, normal, everyday, inexpensive R/S-lipoic acid for the most benefits.

Anyone over the age of forty should take lipoic acid as part of their basic supplement program for its powerful antioxidant properties. For most people, 400 mg a day is sufficient. Clinical studies have used up to 1,000 mg, but only in the short term. Injected lipoic acid is much more effective than oral use, but very impractical, obviously. Overdoses of lipoic acid or anything else merely unbalance our metabolism and are contraindicated. If you have a serious problem, you can safely take 800 mg a day for one year. Take 400 mg in the AM and another 400 mg in the PM to maintain maximum blood levels. Lipoic acid is safe, inexpensive, and non-toxic, but there just isn't any reason to take more than 400 mg for the long term. Short-term studies have used higher doses, but you'll be doing long-term therapy.

THE SCIENCE BEHIND LIPOIC ACID

At Eberhard Karls University in Germany (*BioFactors* v. 10, 1993), a study titled, "Thioctic Acid Effects on Insulin Sensitivity and Glucose Metabolism," was done. They pointed out that, "Thioctic acid is a co-factor of key mitochondrial enzymes, involved in the regulation of glucose oxidation, such as the pyruvate dehydrogenase and the alpha-ketoglutarate dehydrogenase, both enzyme complexes which are known to be diminished in diabetes." In plain words, this means lipoic acid works with our body's enzymes to prevent glucose from being oxidized. Their conclusion was, "The clinical and experimental data indicate that this compound has beneficial effects on insulin sensitivity, correcting several metabolic pathways known to be altered in type 2 diabetes, such as insulin stimulated glucose uptake, glucose oxidation, and glycogen synthesis." The authors quote two human studies published in *Diabetologica* (1995) and *Arzneimittelforschung* (1995). Here insulin sensitivity was increased from 27 percent to 51 percent in merely ten days! This is nothing less than incredible! No dangerous, synthetic, toxic prescription drugs can even start to approach results like that.

At the University of Southern California (*Nutrition* v. 17, 2001), "Molecular Aspects of Lipoic Acid in the Prevention of Diabetes Complications," was published. People with diabetes suffer from an endless list of complications, eventually ending in premature death. These include vascular (heart and artery) disease, cataracts, retinopathy (vision loss), and neuropathy (nerve deterioration). "The available data strongly suggest that LA, because of its antioxidant properties, is particularly suited to the prevention and/or treatment of diabetic complications. In addition to its antioxidant properties, LA increases glucose uptake. Further, recent trials have demonstrated that LA improves glucose disposal in patients with type 2 diabetes. In experimental and clinical studies, LA markedly reduced the symptoms of diabetic pathologies, including cataract formation, vascular damage, and poly-neuropathy." Rather powerful statements from top doctors in the best hospitals.

Reviews are always best. A most impressive seventeen-page, heavily documented review, "The Pharmacology of the Antioxidant Lipoic Acid," from Vrije University in Amsterdam (*General Pharmacology* v. 29, 1997) leaves no doubt about the effectiveness of lipoic acid. Here they prove that the R- and S-isomers equally convert to DHLA in humans. Do not waste your money on R-only lipoic acid. This review is about the antioxidant properties of LA for general health, rather than the benefits for diabetes specifically. The language here is highly technical, and refers to reactive oxygen species (ROS), NADH, chelation, oxidative stress, and other such topics. In plain English, they show LA supplements to be a most powerful and proven antioxidant that has many benefits as we age. It is an important overall anti-aging supplement that everyone over forty needs.

At the University of Arizona (*Oxidative Stress and Disease* v. 8, 2002), a long, well-documented review was done on hyperglycemia and insulin resistance. The researchers strongly suggest using LA as a therapy for both conditions. Further, they discuss the underlying mechanisms for using LA in diabetic and prediabetic conditions, so we can better understand how it is so effective. At Oregon State University (*Current Medicinal Chemistry* v. 11, 2004), a twelve-page review with extensive references was done showing the power of LA to help ameliorate the pathophysiologies of many chronic diseases—not just diabetes—and other forms of blood sugar dysmetabolism. They found lipoic acid therapy to have dramatic benefits in patients in only thirty days. This was true not only for diabetes, but also other diseases associated with oxidative stress. Lipoic acid was found to be an effective agent to improve certain pathophysiologies of many chronic diseases. Here the evidence was examined for the effectiveness of lipoic acid against such diverse age-related disorders, such as unwarranted apoptosis (programmed cell death), cardiovascular disease, and cataract formation. The famous Mayo Clinic in Minnesota did a most impressive sixteen-page review, complete with seventy-seven references (*Antioxidants in Health and Disease* v. 6, 1997) on lipoic acid. This study leaves no doubt as to the proven effectiveness on any disease associated with oxidative stress, including blood sugar disorders in general. At the University of California in Los Angeles, a sophisticated review with an impressive seventy-eight citations (*Toxicology and Applied Pharmacology* v. 182, 2002), was done on the general antioxidant and pro-oxidant properties of lipoic acid. They showed both lipoic acid and dihydrolipoic acid exhibit direct free radical scavenging properties. Other studies provide evidence that lipoic acid supplementation has pro-oxidant properties, decreases oxidative stress, and restores reduced levels of other antioxidants in real people.

Three different reviews were done at the University of California in Berkeley. Another good review, with thirty-four references (*Annals of the NY Academy of Sciences* v. 738, 1994), was done on the properties of lipoic acid in relation to oxidative stress and disease. Another was published in *Environmental & Nutritional Interactions* v. 3, 1999). This thorough twenty-eight page article showed the effectiveness of LA for diabetes itself, as well as the serious complications that come with it. Neuropathy is the worst side effect of diabetes. Many dozens of studies show that LA alone helps relieve the symptoms of mono-, poly-, autonomic and peripheral neuropathy. A third study from *Oxidative Stress and Disease* v. 4, 2000 had thirty-eight references. This demonstrated the dramatic antioxidant effects of LA.

CONCLUSION

Lipoic acid is an important antioxidant that will destroy many of the free radicals that are destructive to the body. It has also been shown to significantly reduce complications associated with diabetes. The studies cited above are just a small fraction of the studies performed that proved the effectiveness of lipoic acid. There are many other published human studies from around the world that promote the supplementation of oral lipoic acid for blood sugar and insulin metabolism. Supplementing your diet with lipoic acid is very important for anyone over the age of forty, or for anyone with a blood sugar level over 85 mg/dL. Make this a part of your supplement program to prevent and cure blood sugar issues.

9. The Minerals You Need

We are all mineral-deficient, every one of us. No matter how well you eat or what supplements you take, you're still lacking in some of the vital elements you need. Every illness is due in part to mineral deficiency of some kind. Our soils are depleted of minerals. Our food lacks minerals. We don't eat well anyway. There are ninety-two natural elements, but modern medicine only recognizes ten of them as essential. This is irrational and defies logic. While sodium, potassium, phosphorous, and sulfur are all essential elements, we get enough of these in our food.

Science has shown how important minerals are for every disease and medical condition. Every single health problem known is due in part to mineral deficiency. Various minerals are helpful in treating diabetes and slowing down diabetic complications. Let's look at the twenty-one elements we are known to need for optimal health (See Table 6.1 on page 51).

BORON

Boron is acknowledged as an essential element, but the RDA has never been set. It was only in 1990 that boron was even accepted as essential! A valid estimate is 3 mg a day, but Americans generally only eat about 1 mg. Our soils are boron-deficient, our food is boron-deficient, and vitamin supplements rarely contain what you need. Boron is necessary for calcium absorption, among many other important processes. You would think that all widely sold vitamin and mineral supplements would contain 3 mg of this inexpensive and vital element, but very few actually do. It must be emphasized how important it is to get boron in your diet every day. Our soils and foods are very deficient. You cannot absorb calcium without sufficient boron. The published research here is overwhelming.

DOSAGE: Take 3 mg a day of boron. Any common salt such as citrate, or even plain boric acid is fine.

CALCIUM

Calcium is very misunderstood. The idea that we need 1,000 mg a day is ridiculous, and the official government RDA is not based on science whatsoever. The only abundant source of calcium is dairy products, and at least two-thirds of the world's population does not include dairy foods in their diet. Billions of Asians prove this. You cannot possibly get 1,000 mg of calcium a day without eating dairy foods. You should not eat dairy foods because of the lactose (milk sugar) and casein content. All adults of all races are lactose intolerant. Americans and Europeans eat more calcium than anyone on earth, yet they have the highest rates of bone and joint disease, especially arthritis and osteoporosis. Obviously, calcium intake isn't the problem, but rather calcium absorption. You need, at minimum, magnesium, boron, silicon, strontium, omega-3s, and vitamin D in order to absorb the calcium. You aren't getting enough of these nutrients. There are certainly other nutritional factors in calcium absorption we haven't discovered yet.

DOSAGE: Taking 250 mg a day of any common, inexpensive calcium salts such as citrates and carbonates is sufficient. Overdosing on calcium is irresponsible and won't benefit you. More is not better.

CESIUM

Cesium has no RDA, but it is certainly essential. This ultra-trace element has proven value from extensive research, especially in human blood. It is almost impossible to find in any supplements. A reasonable dose is 100 mcg, although irresponsible promoters have been recommending much larger, toxic quantities that supposedly cure cancer and "alkalinize" the body.

DOSAGE: This is an ultra-trace element, and 100 mcg is an ideal dose.

CHROMIUM

Chromium has dozens of published studies, and the research is most impressive, showing that people with diabetes usually have deficient levels. This is due to a lack of chromium in their food. It must always be emphasized that we need *all* the known essential elements, and not just ones like chromium that are proven to benefit glucose metabolism. Again, whole grains are the best source, and the refined grains we eat lack any significant amounts. You can take inexpensive chelates (a metal ion bound to non-metal ions) here. Do not listen to advertisements telling you that a certain patented form is the "best" or "only" form that works. The research on chromium and blood sugar metabolism is overwhelming. This must be in your supplement program.

DOSAGE: The RDA is 120 mcg. This is toxic in high amounts, so don't exceed 400 mcg.

COBALT

Cobalt is a very neglected element, although it is the central atom for chlorophyll in plants and vitamin B_{12} in animals. Humans cannot synthesize B_{12} without available cobalt, and oral vitamin B_{12} supplements are barely absorbed. (Use 1 mg of methyl cobalamin as your B_{12} source.) This is a very important ultra-trace element, even though it is needed in such tiny amounts. Almost no mineral supplements contain cobalt.

DOSAGE: We probably only need about 25 mcg of cobalt a day, but it is not toxic and you could certainly take up to 100 mcg.

COPPER

Copper levels vary greatly in diabetics; some have low blood levels, while others have high levels. Americans only get about half of the RDA of 2 mg in their food. Whole grains and beans are the best source. Our bodies contain a total of only about 150 mg. Anything over 15 mg daily could cause side effects, as it is a heavy element. It is almost impossible to get excessive copper in your diet, even with copper water pipes in your home. Inexpensive salts such as citrates, gluconates, or oxides are very bioavailable.

DOSAGE: Copper has an RDA of 2 mg. Common salts such as citrates, oxides, or gluconates are good.

GALLIUM

Gallium is an important, but ignored, ultra-trace element. Human blood studies, as well as animal and food studies prove this is essential. It is found in all our organs. The earth's crust has an amazing 10 mg per kg of gallium. A Japanese study showed that people are taking in a mere 12 mcg a day. Other human blood and organ studies indicate common deficiency.

DOSAGE: Taking 100 mcg per day of gallium nitrate is a good dose.

GERMANIUM

Germanium is something you almost never find in any vitamin-mineral supplement. There is no RDA here. Science has proven this is, in fact, essential, as it is an ultra-trace element. In 1988, a very impressive review was published in the journal *Medical Hypothesis*, complete with seventy-two references. This showed the importance of germanium in human and animal nutrition. Very irresponsible promoters offer 100 mg (100,000 mcg) doses. This is 1,000 times what you need—a three-year supply every day. You will almost never find a supplement with 100 mcg of germanium for a complete minerals program. This is an essential element for optimal health.

DOSAGE: Taking 100 mcg per day is a good dose. Germanium sesquioxide is safe, but germanium dioxide is not.

IODINE

Iodine is most needed for thyroid metabolism. There are only about 30 mg (30,000 mcg) of iodine in your body, and three-fourths of this is in your thyroid gland. If you have low T3 (triiodothyronine) or low T4 (L-thyroxine), you should take bioidentical hormones to raise them. Iodine supplements will *not* raise your hormone levels. Seaweed and kelp are the best sources, but the problem here is that they are *too* good. While Asians often eat sea vegetables as a staple, a mere teaspoon of kelp powder can contain twenty times the RDA. This can cause side effects such as skin problems. Megadoses of any mineral are clearly not advised. You do not need iodized salt, by the way.

DOSAGE: The RDA is 150 mcg, and most mineral supplements have this.

IRON

Iron is very important, as it is the "heme" in blood hemoglobin. Women need more than men, and studies consistently show that Americans are generally iron-deficient, especially women, vegetarians, and the elderly. People with diabetes may have a problem excreting iron and end up with excessive blood levels of it. This is a rare condition, which is not due to excessive intake, but rather an inability to get rid of unneeded iron. Just be careful not to take more than 18 mg a day. Studies also prove iron from animal foods is the real culprit. Again, diabetics often show a problem with iron retention and high blood ferritin (iron) levels.

DOSAGE: Men need about 10 mg a day, and women need about 18 mg. Common inexpensive salts such as sulfates, fumarates, and gluconates are good.

MAGNESIUM

Magnesium is the most studied and most important element in preventing and curing diabetes. Magnesium is vitally important for our total health since we're generally deficient in it. One in seven Americans is seriously deficient according to blood analysis studies. The major source of magnesium is whole grains, yet almost all of the grain we eat is refined. Americans only eat 1-percent whole grains. There is overwhelming evidence that magnesium is critical to blood sugar and insulin metabolism, as well as outright diabetes.

DOSAGE: The RDA is 400 mg, so taking 200 mg per day is good. Citrates, lactates, or oxides are good choices.

MANGANESE

Manganese has overwhelming research on it for its value in human and animal nutrition. Many people do, in fact, get that much in their food. Whole grains, beans, and leafy vegetables are the best sources. We only have about 20 mg of manganese in our entire bodies.

DOSAGE: The RDA was only recently set at 2 mg. You can take any normal form, such as sulfates or oxides.

MOLYBDENUM

Molybdenum has an official RDA of 75 mcg, but some scientists feel this is too low. This is in most vitamin-mineral supplements. Inexpensive common salts are good sources. Molybdenum is safe and non-toxic, even though it is a very heavy metal. Research on molybdenum is extensive and goes back decades. Progressive farmers use this to fertilize their soils, and ranchers use it to insure the health of their livestock.

DOSAGE: Deficiency is not widespread here, but taking a mere 75 mcg a day is good insurance, especially since dietary intake varies so greatly.

NICKEL

Nickel has no RDA but is definitely an essential element. The published research has concentrated on animals rather than humans. The few human studies we have are most impressive, however. You'll almost never find meaningful amounts in any supplements, so look for one with 100 mcg.

DOSAGE: This is an ultra-trace element, and 100 mcg per day would be a reasonable dosage based on various analyses of human dietary intake and blood analyses.

RUBIDIUM

Rubidium has no RDA, is not a mere trace element, and is definitely essential. Why is an element that is needed in such large amounts and found in large amounts in common foods misnamed a "trace" element? Rubidium is very ignored for some reason. No deficiency has been shown for this, however. This is found rather abundantly in common foods.

DOSAGE: Taking 500 mcg per day is a reasonable dose.

SELENIUM

Selenium has an official RDA of 70 mcg, which was only recently established. Deficiency is common, because the main source is whole grains, and most all our grains are heavily refined. Chelates are the best form here. This is a very important antioxidant element, as it fights free radicals. Studies have shown that people with low selenium intake have more cancer, heart and artery disease, diabetes, and other illnesses. Generally, most vitamin formulas contain the 70 mcg you need.

DOSAGE: Taking 200 IU of natural mixed tocopherol (vitamin E) per day works synergistically and helps selenium metabolism. Do not take more than 200 mcg per day, as toxicity can occur in doses higher than over this amount. It is a heavy metal and will accumulate in the body if overdoses are used.

SILICON

Silicon is a vital yet ignored element with no set RDA, even though it has been proven essential in human and animal health. You will almost never find this in any vitamin supplement. Silicon levels in common foods vary greatly, so it is hard to be more precise. One major need for silicon (not to be confused with silicone, which is a polymer of silicon and oxygen) is for bone and joint metabolism, and calcium absorption. Why aren't vitamin companies putting this inexpensive essential element in their formulas? Be sure to get silicon in your mineral supplement.

DOSAGE: A good dose is 10 mg per day, although you probably don't need that much. It isn't toxic, so 10 mg is a safe and effective amount. Plain silica gel (silicic acid) is the best form to take. Do not use horsetail herb. Make sure the label says silicic acid.

STRONTIUM

Strontium has no RDA, but it is definitely essential and needed for calcium absorption. Do not confuse this with radioactive strontium-90. Food and blood analysis studies around the world show that 1,000 mcg (1 mg) a day is certainly enough. Doctors prescribing 250 mg of strontium ranelate is outright insanity. Make sure this is in your supplement.

DOSAGE: A good dose would be 1,000 mcg (1 mg) a day. A chelate or aspartate is a good choice. There is no need to take more than this, although some irresponsible natural health "experts" recommend much more.

TIN

Tin has no RDA, but it is definitely an essential ultra-trace element. The same comments about research on nickel apply to that of tin. Human research has found low tin levels in various pathological conditions and diseases. We need more human research on tin. You'll almost never find meaningful amounts in any of the supplements currently in the marketplace.

DOSAGE: A reasonable dosage is 100 mcg per day, but the FDA irrationally limits this to 30 mcg per day.

VANADIUM

Vanadium has finally been accepted as an essential element (not a mere trace element), but no RDA has been set. There has been an overwhelming amount of research on blood sugar metabolism and vanadium in the last decade. Scientists around the world have studied this for diabetes and Syndrome X in dozens of published studies and reviews. While there is no RDA, a daily dose of 1,000 mcg (1 mg) is sufficient. It is not a good idea to take more than this, although short-term studies have used more. Using more than 1 mg is very irresponsible, and will result in vanadium toxicity eventually. Therefore, vanadium becomes overemphasized as a diabetes mineral, and the other supporting minerals that work with it are ignored. You will almost never find this in vitamin supplements. This must be in your supplement program, as it is proven to be essential, not only for blood sugar metabolism, but also your general health.

DOSAGE: Take only 1 mg daily. Inexpensive chelates or vanadyl sulfate are both good choices.

ZINC

Zinc is also generally deficient in our diets. Again, whole grains and beans are the primary source, yet what little grains we do eat are almost all refined with the nutrition removed. Eating whole grains and beans (legumes) every day will go a long way in raising your levels. The elderly, the poor, and people who drink alcohol have the lowest levels generally. The problem in diabetes is poor zinc metabolism, rather than deficient zinc intake. There are many clinical studies showing poor zinc metabolism in people with blood sugar conditions. Common inexpensive salts such as citrates, sulfates, and oxides are good.

DOSAGE: The RDA is 15 mg. You have to be careful not to take too much zinc, as amounts over 50 mg can cause side effects. This is a heavy metal and can accumulate in the body.

OTHER ULTRA-TRACE ELEMENTS

Let's talk about other essential and possibly essential ultra-trace elements. *Tungsten* is definitely needed. *Barium* is definitely essential. *Lithium* is definitely essential, but we seem to get sufficient amounts in our food. Doctors giving people 1,000 times the needed amount for depression is irresponsible and very dangerous. *Titanium* has evidence showing it to be essential. *Europium* seems to be essential, and research will probably validate this within the next ten years. *Lanthanum* has considerable research behind it and is probably essential. *Indium* is claimed to have numerous benefits on Internet sites, but published research simply doesn't verify any of this. *Neodymium* has shown potential in animal as well as human metabolism. *Thulium* (not thallium) has soil and edible plant studies to indicate its importance, and animal studies will soon tell us more. *Praseodymium* has some animal and human research that indicates value for our health. *Gandolium* may also be shown to be essential eventually. *Samarium* is found in our blood in significant amounts. *Yttrium* may be essential. *Cerium* has evidence it may be needed. *Erbium* is found in our blood and food. *Dysprosium* may be essential as well.

CONCLUSION

We need all the known essential elements and not just some of them. All elements work synergistically and harmoniously together, in concert, as a team. You must get *all* of them, and not just some of them. We know there are at least twenty-one we need. Search the Internet under "mineral supplements" to find a comprehensive one that includes most or all of the ones discussed in this chapter. Read the label, and look at the amounts contained in the product.

10. Your Basic Hormones

Insulin is the primary hormone involved in glucose metabolism, but it is only one of our basic hormones (twelve in men and fifteen in women). We should understand that all hormones work together synergistically in concert, together in harmony as a team, just like minerals. People with blood sugar dysmetabolism generally have been shown to have other hormones out of balance. It is important that you try to balance all your basic hormones. You want to strive for the youthful, ideal hormone levels you had at age thirty. You do not want "normal" levels found for older people. In the next chapter, we'll talk about your basic hormones, and how to test them with blood and saliva.

As with minerals, if one member of the team isn't doing well, all the other players are strongly affected. It is of little value to balance a few of your hormones, and ignore the others. All your basic hormones must be balanced as much as possible in order for them to work together harmoniously. Men and women have exactly the same hormones, only in different amounts. Let's briefly discuss the fourteen basic human hormones.

ANDROSTENEDIONE

Androstenedione levels generally parallel testosterone, since this hormone and androstenediol are the direct precursors to testosterone in our bodies. You generally do not have to measure this or supplement with it. If a woman has high testosterone or DHEA, it would be a good idea to test her androstenedione as well. The only way to lower hyper levels in women (again, men do not have hyper levels) is by diet, exercise, and balancing the other basic hormones. Androstenedione was classified as a prescription drug in 2004, and is now a felony to possess or sell.

CORTISOL

Cortisol is the stress hormone. Researchers agree that diabetics tend to have higher levels of cortisol. High levels indicate an inability to deal with stress on a daily basis. The ideal way to measure this is a 24-hour, four-sample diagnosis at 9/1/5/9. If you have high cortisol, you must eat better, take supplements, balance your other hormones, exercise, and somehow deal with the factors causing stress in your life. Deficient levels are unusual, but Cortef can be taken at the exact time your level is low. You really don't need to bother with cortisol at all. This is completely optional. Cortisol is what it is.

DHEA

DHEA is the third androgen. This is very much a life extension hormone, and critical to your health and longevity. Studies again show that diabetic men are usually deficient, while women can be too low or too high. Men rarely have excessive levels, while women sometimes have too much DHEA. As always, you are looking for the youthful level you had at age thirty. If low, women can take half-tablets (12.5 mg) of DHEA orally, and men can take the regular 25-mg tablets. Never use DHEA unless you have proven by blood or saliva analyses that you are low. This is a very powerful hormone, and excessive levels are harmful. Some men will find they cannot metabolize oral DHEA and are androgen resistant. Transdermal creams are *not* effective here because of the poor absorption. Injections are neither practical nor natural. DHEA (and pregnenolone) is only about 10 percent absorbed orally. Do not use expensive "7-keto DHEA," as it has no science behind it.

ESTRADIOL

Estradiol (E2) is the strongest, and potentially the most dangerous, of the three basic estrogens. Most American women are up to their ears in estradiol and estrone. Men over fifty generally have more estradiol and estrone than their postmenopausal wives.

Only diet and lifestyle will lower hyper estradiol levels, not toxic prescription drugs. Very, very few women will need supplementary estradiol. Low normal values much preferred here. Westerners generally have excessive levels. Vegetarians and rural Asians have lower levels. All females of any age, with even mild gynecological problems, should test all three estrogen levels. Patches are expensive, oral pills are not absorbed well, transdermal creams deliver only about 20 percent, sublingual drops are almost unknown (but most effective), and DMSO solutions not approved by the FDA. Transdermal creams and sublingual drops can be prepared by a compounding pharmacist if you get a prescription. A good dose is 50 mcg a day in the blood. Estradiol is very powerful and should be used only by women who are actually low *out* of range. This is rare to find.

ESTRIOL

Estriol (E3), like pregnenolone, is another "orphan" hormone. This has very little research available, especially when compared with estradiol and estrone. Common sense tells you that women must maintain youthful estriol levels. Men do not need to test this. Estriol comprises about 80 percent of human estrogen, and is the "good" or beneficial estrogen. Doctors do not measure estriol or prescribe it. Normal pharmacies do not carry it! Only a compounding pharmacist can supply it legally, but it is still available on the Internet inexpensively. Get a 0.25 percent transdermal cream or gel (150 mg per 2-ounce jar), and use a half-gram a day. Sublingual drops in oil should contain about 500 mcg per drop. Vaginal gels are effective, but are inconvenient and unnecessary. Never use oral tablets, as they are very ineffective. If a blood or saliva test shows you are low, you want to deliver about 500 mcg a day into your blood. Strive for high normal ranges here, since rural Asian women and vegetarians have higher levels.

ESTRONE

Estrone (E1) is the second basic estrogen. The same information and advice equally applies, as with estradiol. Estrone is not as powerful as estradiol, but is still very potent. High levels cause a wide range of health problems. For the few women who are actually low (out of range) in estrone, they can use transdermal creams or sublingual drops, as with estradiol. Look to deliver about 100 mcg a day into your blood. Very few women are low in this, so supplementation is rarely needed.

GROWTH HORMONE

Growth hormone (GH) is the most expensive hormone of all, because it is difficult to make such a complex 191-amino acid chain molecule. Just because GH is expensive, does not mean that it is any more important than other hormones, or that you will get any more dramatic effects. GH metabolism is disrupted in blood sugar conditions, and patients can have low, normal, or even high levels. You just cannot generalize here. The Chinese produce inexpensive GH for about $120 or less a month (30 IU). This is a tightly controlled prescription drug. Any HGH product you see sold over the counter is worthless, especially homeopathic GH and GH "secretagogues." You can legally buy this on the Internet from online pharmacies for your own personal use, but most of these have been shut down. You need to inject this subcutaneously (under your skin, or s.c.). Sublingual GH in DMSO works well but is not legal. One milligram equals three international units. The average adult needs 1 IU (0.33 mg) a day. It is very difficult to blood test GH levels, and GH rises dramatically—about 1,000 percent (ten times)—around midnight, after you go to sleep. You cannot saliva test for this, and IGF-1 levels do not parallel GH levels, despite the "conventional wisdom." You need to go by actual results here. Just go by real world results, rather than by blood testing. Do not even think of using GH until all your other basic hormones are balanced. This is a very overrated hormone. Are you willing to spend $1,500 a year on this? Think twice before buying this supplement.

INSULIN

Insulin can be measured directly, but few people should measure theirs directly. The glucose tolerance test (GTT) is much more informative, as it tells the *response* of the insulin to a sugar load. The *response* of insulin is more important than the blood levels per se. The GTT test is excellent, inexpensive, and very underused. Because of the epidemic of insulin resistance and other blood sugar conditions, a GTT should be a routine part of a yearly physical, rather than measuring insulin per se. You want to be at least ten points below the accepted healthy level. If you have a fasting blood sugar level of 85 mg/dL of less, you probably don't need a GTT. Do not accept the usual figure of 100 mg/dL or less as it just isn't good enough. Fasting blood sugar is a very accurate indicator, and if yours is over 85 mg/dL, get a GTT test.

MELATONIN

Melatonin is a powerful antioxidant hormone. Melatonin is much more powerful and beneficial than the media tells you, and has even been studied for cancer therapy. Even though levels fall from the time we are eighteen, it is best you test your melatonin level if you are over the age of forty. You cannot assume you are low just because you are older. Hyper levels are medically unknown (except rarely with pineal tumors). A few people are melatonin-deficient throughout life and would ben-

efit from early diagnosis. We have discussed the vital importance of antioxidants and oxidative stress in blood sugar conditions. This is a very underestimated hormone, despite numerous
published studies showing major benefits in real people (including immunity enhancement and antioxidant properties) for
many diseases. Men over forty can take 3 mg at night, and
women, half-tablets (1.5 mg). Only take this at night, when levels naturally rise, and never during the day. Taking this during
the day would produce negative effects. You can only test melatonin at 3:00 AM with a saliva test kit.

There are literally dozens of valid animal studies proving
the benefit of youthful melatonin levels for diabetes and blood
sugar disorders. We are now getting many human studies. At
Granada University in Spain (*Journal of Pineal Research* v. 35,
2003), both blood and saliva testing showed diabetics to be
about 40 percent lower in melatonin. Here, age-matched type 1
and type 2 patients of both sexes were used. Plasma melatonin
averaged only 8.98 pg/mL in patients, but 14.91 in healthy controls. This is most impressive, since both type 1 and 2, as well as
both men and women patients, were used. More human studies
on melatonin will be forthcoming, not only for diabetes, but also
many other chronic illnesses.

PREGNENOLONE

Pregnenolone is the "orphan" hormone, like estriol. There is very
little research, despite its great importance to our health and
well-being. Studies on pregnenolone and diabetes are almost
non-existent. This is the "grandmother" hormone from which
all the other sex hormones are derived. Pregnenolone is the
brain and cognition hormone. Our levels fall at about the age of
thirty-five to forty and then stabilize. Despite the lack of research
here, you must balance your pregnenolone level so that all your
other hormones can work effectively. Men over forty can take 50
mg if they prove to be low, and women, about 25 mg. There are
no saliva kits in 2012, and doctors will overcharge you to test

this. Go to websites such as www.walkinclinic.com to test this without a doctor. You are looking for the youthful level you had at age thirty, as always. This will help keep your mind, memory, and cognition strong in your elderly years. This is the most important brain, memory, and cognition hormone of all. Use this with PS and ALC (see pages 42 and 47).

PROGESTERONE

Progesterone is not just a "female" hormone, although it is derived from "pro-gestation." Buy a product with about 1,000 mg per 2-ounce jar. Many women of any age can benefit here. Saliva testing does *not* work well, since it is fat soluble. You can measure this with blood according to your monthly cycle. After menopause it doesn't matter, of course, when you measure it. Postmenopausal women can safely use this during any two weeks of the month without testing, since their ovaries no longer produce this. Men can use one-eighth of a teaspoon five days a week directly on their scrotums to protect against excess estrogens as they age. Progesterone is therefore *anti-feminizing* in men. Men need youthful levels of progesterone just as women do.

TESTOSTERONE

Testosterone is not the "male hormone" at all, even though men have about ten times as much as women. Men and women both need youthful levels of this primary androgen. Men cannot have hyper levels, as the testes cannot overproduce this. Even if men over-supplement with testosterone, the excess basically spills over into estradiol and estrone. Overdoses just make estrogens in men. Literally over 90 percent of men over the age of fifty have low testosterone and would benefit from supplementation. Women have only about one-tenth of the blood testosterone that men have, but they can have deficient or excessive levels. Hyper levels in women can be lowered only by diet and lifestyle, not dangerous prescription drugs. A high level of testosterone, androstenedione, and/or DHEA in women is called "andro-genicity." This is a hallmark of polycystic ovaries—a very common condition. Studies repeatedly show diabetic men generally have deficient levels, while women generally have excessive ones. Doctors generally have no idea how to accurately measure testosterone, much less administer it. They usually prescribe dangerous injections, toxic oral salts, or overpriced patches and weak gels. Transdermal creams or gels of natural testosterone, and sublingual tablets or drops of testosterone enanthate are the preferred methods. (Natural testosterone tastes terrible.) Transdermal creams and gels generally only deliver 20 percent into the blood, so 80 percent is wasted. DMSO solutions deliver about 98 percent, are safe and effective, but are not allowed under FDA regulations. Nor are nasal sprays. Men make about 6 to 8 mg a day, so they generally need only about a 3 mg (3,000 mcg) daily dose in their blood. This means a man would use a daily 4-mg sublingual tablet or drops of a salt (containing 3 mg actual testosterone). A woman would use a daily 200-mcg sublingual tablet or drops of a salt (containing 150 mg of actual testosterone). Women make about 300 mcg a day, so about 150 mcg in their blood is a good daily dose, since they store testosterone more efficiently. If a man gets a 100-g tube of 3 percent natural (3 g per 100 g) cream, each half gram will have 15 mg. He can expect 3 mg (20 percent) to actually go into his blood. The tube will therefore last for over six months (200 days). If a woman gets a 100-g tube of a mere 0.15 percent natural (150 mg per 100 g) cream each half-gram will contain 750 mcg. She can expect 150 mcg (20 percent) to go into her blood. Men who are "androgen resistant," and cannot use testosterone or DHEA, simply cannot use any androgen, as they will just get estrogens. Even pregnenolone, nandrolone, HCG, aspartic acid, and other testosterone boosters will spill over into estrogens in such cases. Even aromatase inhibitors, like formestane and ATD will eventually just turn into estrogens. There is no known cure and no research being done here.

T3 AND T4

T3 *(triiodothyronine)* and T4 *(L-thyroxine)* are your two thyroid hormones. Thyroid metabolism is generally slow in both type 1 and 2 diabetics. Get an inexpensive blood test for these. Test your free T3 and free T4. Do *not* let the doctor test the traditional TSH and T3 uptake; these do not accurately indicate thyroid function. Again, you must test your free T3 and free T4, regardless of what your doctor tells you. You can use websites like www.healthcheckusa.com to get this done inexpensively. Doctors know little about thyroid diagnosis, and this includes endocrinologists. Here you cannot accept low normal values, even though they are technically "in range." You need mid-range or better values. Add high and low ranges and divide by 2. T3 and T4 are both bioidentical hormones, with no side effects whatsoever when used properly. That's right—Synthroid and Cytomel are exactly the same as the hormones in your body. Do not use Armour Thyroid from pigs, as it contains a 4:1 ratio of T4 and T3. Very few people (i.e. 5 percent) are low in both. Treat T3 and T4 separately. For people with excessive levels, only diet and lifestyle will lower them; do not get surgery or irradiate your thyroid gland!

CONCLUSION

The hormones covered throughout this chapter are all vital in order for your body to function properly. Each of the basic hormones provides significant health benefits. When these hormones are imbalanced, they may affect our blood sugar levels. Remember to regularly test your hormone levels so that you can maintain a healthy hormone balance. In the next chapter, we will learn how to test our hormones without a doctor.

11. Hormone Testing

Currently, the medical profession is in the Dark Ages when it comes to basic hormone testing. This includes endocrinologists, who are supposed to specialize in the diagnosis and treatment of hormonal balance. Even the most prominent diabetes specialists simply have no idea that all the basic hormones should be balanced in order to successfully treat and cure blood sugar problems. Their only concern is insulin!

Balancing your basic hormones really can be very simple, inexpensive, and straightforward, as you have already seen in the previous chapter. Fortunately, you can test most of your hormones at home with saliva test kits for less than thirty dollars. Saliva testing has been used successfully for decades in clinical settings. It is only in the last decade that it has been offered to the general public. You simply send your saliva sample to a diagnostic lab for RIA (radioimmunoassay) testing. Saliva always gives free, bio-available hormone levels, and never bound unavailable ones. You can readily find such testing services on the Internet by typing in "saliva hormone testing," "hormone testing," and similar terms on your favorite search engine.

ANDROSTENEDIONE

Men don't need to test androstenedione, but women should if they have either a high DHEA and/or testosterone level. All three of these hormones are "androgens." Women who have hyper levels of any or all of these suffer from such problems as polycystic ovary syndrome (PCOS) and hirsutism (hair growth). Androstenedione levels generally parallel those of testosterone.

CORTISOL

Cortisol is the stress hormone and can be tested with saliva. You can buy a saliva kit and take four different saliva samples in a twelve-hour period at 9/1/5/9. Only diet, exercise, and lifestyle will help you lower cortisol. Hypocortisol (low) levels are uncommon, but you can take bioidentical cortisol (oral hydro-cortisone) known as Cortef supplements if you have this problem. You really don't need to bother with cortisol testing at all. Spend your time and effort on your other hormones.

DHEA

Test your DHEA or DHEA-S (sulfate) with either a saliva kit or a blood draw. Look for the youthful level you had at the age of thirty. Remember that people, especially women, can suffer from hyper levels, which are just as harmful as hypo levels. DHEA levels generally fall as we age, especially after the age of forty.

ESTRADIOL, ESTRONE, AND ESTRIOL

Teenage girls, as well as premenopausal and postmenopausal women, should all test their estradiol, estrone, and estriol levels with a saliva kit according to their cycle. Men don't need to do this unless they are using testosterone supplements (which can aromatize into estradiol and estrone) or suspect any kind of hormonal imbalance, such as prostate problems and gynecomastia. Doctors, including endocrinologists, do not test for or prescribe estriol, nor is it sold in normal pharmacies. Doctors blindly prescribe dangerous oral estradiol and estrone supplements to women without even testing their levels.

GROWTH HORMONE

Growth hormone (GH) cannot currently be tested with saliva. It is difficult to test with a blood draw due to the fact it varies a lot during the day. This must be tested in a clinic with four blood draws, say at 9/1/5/9 in one day. It is best to go by real world results here. Just go by actual physical results you get from supplementation. If you are over fifty, your GH levels are surely low, and you could benefit somewhat from taking it. You would have to inject 1 IU (0.33 mg) s.c. (subcutaneously) every day, or use it sublingually in DMSO. Do not even consider taking GH until all your other basic hormones are balanced. This is a very expensive vanity that must be injected daily. It will cost at least $1,500 a year for a Chinese prescription, and $3,600 for an American prescription. GH is highly overrated and overpriced.

INSULIN

Rather than test your insulin per se, it is better to get a glucose tolerance test (GTT). You drink a 75-gram measured cup of glucose, wait an hour, and have your blood sugar level tested with a blood draw. If the accepted range is 140 mg, use 120 to130 mg as the more healthful range. Just go 10 to 20 points under the "accepted" level. Make sure your fasting glucose level is 85 mg/dL or less; do not accept the accepted "normal" limit of 100 mg/dL or more. It must be 85 mg/dL or less. The GTT test is inexpensive, accurate, and should be routine for anyone with symptoms of metabolic syndrome and anyone over the age of forty. This is an underutilized tool.

MELATONIN

Your melatonin must be tested at 3:00 AM with a saliva kit. The only other way is to pay a fortune to stay overnight in a sleep lab and get a blood draw. Look for the level you had at the age of thirty. Doctors have no interest in testing or prescribing melatonin, since they don't understand how important it is. Also, it is sold over the counter, so there is no profit in it for them. Our melatonin levels fall from the time we're eighteen until they almost disappear by our seventies. Mostly everyone over forty would benefit from melatonin supplementation. Don't assume you are low just because you are getting older.

PREGNENOLONE

Pregnenolone is the forgotten or orphan hormone, and doctors don't even know what it is or care. Yes, this includes endocrinologists generally. There is almost no research done on pregnenolone, amazingly enough. No saliva tests are available in 2012. Test this with a blood draw at www.walkinclinic.com without a doctor. Look for the level you had at the age of thirty. Levels fall at about the age of thirty-five to forty and then tend to stabilize. Hyper levels are rare. Again, don't assume you are low just because you are getting older. Everyone is biologically unique.

PROGESTERONE

Premenopausal women can test their progesterone levels with blood according to their cycle, and use transdermal progesterone if they are low. This includes teenage girls and women under forty. Testing is optional. Saliva testing just doesn't work well here, since progesterone won't dissolve in water. Postmenopausal women can simply use progesterone for any two weeks of the calendar month, since their ovaries are no longer active. Men over forty should use small amounts of transdermal progesterone (i.e. one-eighth of a teaspoon five days a week), but they don't need to test their levels.

TESTOSTERONE

Test your free testosterone, not your total or bound testosterone. You can do this with a saliva kit or with a blood draw. If you get a blood test, you must explain to the doctor that you do not want your total or bound levels tested, and that you're not interested in any meaningless bound-to-free ratios. Look for the youthful level you had at the age of thirty, not the level that is "normal" for your age. Women must do this even though they only have one-tenth the amount men do. Literally 90 percent of men over the age of fifty are deficient. Women can have hyper or hypo levels.

T3 AND T4

The medical profession is really walking in darkness when it comes to thyroid testing. Doctors will usually waste your time and money testing your TSH (thyroid-stimulating hormone) and T3 uptake, instead of your free T3 and free T4. As of 2012, there is no saliva testing offered, but this situation should change due to demand. Getting your free T3 and free T4 tested is very inexpensive and costs only about thirty dollars for each test, plus the office visit. Go in at about 9:00 AM fasting. Fortunately you can go to websites (like www. healthcheckusa.com) and get this done for under one hundred dollars without a doctor. Do *not* settle for low normal ranges here, but look for mid-range levels. Add high and low ranges and divide by two. Ranges differ from lab to lab; there is no universal range. If you are low, good starting doses are 100 mcg of T4 and 25 mcg of T3 (it is always a 4:1 ratio). You can get bioidential T3 (Cytomel) and T4 (Synthroid) legally on the Internet from Mexican online pharmacies. Search for generic Levoxyl and Cynomel. Do *not* use Armour pig thyroid, as it contains both in a 4:1 ratio, and few (about 5 percent) people need that.

CONCLUSION

Saliva hormone testing kits should be sold in every pharmacy, drug store, and health food store, but surprisingly they are not. You can readily find sources on the Internet by searching for "saliva hormone test" or "saliva hormone testing" using your favorite search engine. There are also now more and more Internet sites offering real blood testing without a doctor. You will never have optimal health until your basic hormones are in balance.

12. Heart Disease and Cholesterol

We need a separate chapter on blood fats and cardiovascular health, because these factors are closely related to blood sugar conditions. One of the hallmarks of Syndrome X and other blood sugar conditions is high total cholesterol (TC) and triglyceride levels. This is called *dyslipidemia*. High triglycerides are more important than total cholesterol levels here. The cholesterol-to-LDL ratio is also important. Divide your total cholesterol by your HDL level, and you should get a ratio of 4.0 or less for men, and 4.5 or less for women. Low HDL and high LDL levels are characteristic of blood sugar conditions generally. The average adult American has an average cholesterol level of about 240. A healthy, good level is about 150, no matter what age, race, or sex you are. Lower cholesterol levels are easily obtainable by simply reducing or cutting out meat, eggs, poultry, and eliminating all dairy products from your diet. Even those genetically predisposed to higher TC levels can easily keep them under 200 with diet and lifestyle. Keep your triglycerides well under 100. C-reactive protein, or CRP, is a very accurate indication of CHD (coronary heart disease) health, and should be under 1.0 mg. Homocysteine is another very accurate blood sugar and CHD indicator, and should be less than 10 mmol. Uric acid is a very accurate test for both blood sugar and CHD, and should be under 5 mg. Keep your total cholesterol, triglycerides, HDL, LDL, c-reactive protein, uric acid, and homocysteine at healthy levels naturally, safely, and effectively without resorting to toxic, dangerous drugs, which can have many negative side effects.

LOWERING BLOOD FATS

Researchers around the world agree that both type 1 and 2 diabetes, insulin resistance, and impaired glucose metabolism are highly correlated with dyslipidemia. There is no reason to review this overwhelming research, as the scientists of the world are in basic agreement on this issue. Our emphasis will therefore be on practical and effective ways to lower our blood fats naturally. Diet is the most important of course. Proven supplements, especially beta-sitosterol, flax oil, beta glucan, and soy isoflavones are the second means. Natural hormone balance is the third, and regular exercise is the fourth. Fasting once a week on water, from dinner to dinner, will also help you lower blood fats.

Supplements will help you only if you eat well. The most important supplement is 300 to 600 mg of beta-sitosterol. Beta-sitosterol is found in literally every vegetable you eat. The studies on lowering blood fats with mixed plant sterols go back over three decades. Most Americans eat only about 300 mg a day, and vegetarians eat about twice that much. We eat too many omega-6 fatty acids and not enough omega-3s. Flax oil is the best known source of omega-3 fatty acids and lignans, and a better choice than fish oil for many reasons. Choose flax oil! Our food is very deficient in omega-3s and very excessive in omega-6s. Beta glucan is the third supplement. Beta glucan is the most powerful immune enhancer known to science, and that includes prescription drugs such as interferon alpha. Beta glucan has also shown effectiveness in lowering blood lipids. People of all ages will benefit from taking 200 mg or more of beta glucan a day. Isoflavones are the fourth supplement. Taking 40 mg of mixed daidzein and genistein soy isoflavones is the most practical and realistic way to get the benefits of soybeans. Western people simply don't eat enough soy foods to get sufficient isoflavones in their diet. Soy foods just aren't a part of Western culture.

CHOLESTEROL

Pseudo-experts who tell you that cholesterol is not an important indicator of CHD health and longevity prove their complete lack of knowledge in this area. It has become faddish to say "cholesterol doesn't count," so people have an excuse to continue their high fat diets. Some frauds go even further and tell you that low cholesterol is somehow "dangerous." Many elderly people are so sickly that they lose their ability to manufacture cholesterol, despite a high fat diet. Therefore, their lower cholesterol levels are *not* indicative of good health at all, but rather of morbidity. The chart below, which is from the Multiple Risk Factor Intervention Trial (MRFIT), proves beyond any doubt that total cholesterol should ideally be about 150 mg/dL. A total of 361,662

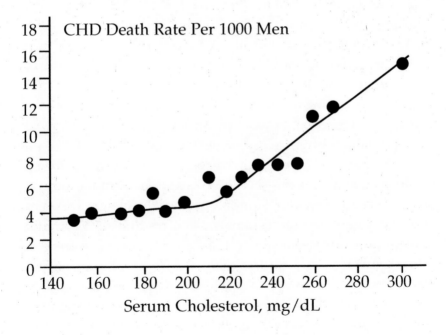

Figure 12.1 The MRFIT Study

men from forty different countries and between the ages of thirty-five and fifty-seven, (*Archives of Internal Medicine* v. 148, 1998) were studied over a period of six years. The ones with low cholesterol had only three deaths per thousand every year, while the ones with high cholesterol had sixteen deaths per thousand annually. That is 533 percent more deaths. They summarized this as, "The association between serum cholesterol and six year risk of CHD was continuous, graded, and strong over the entire range . . ."

The famous Seven Countries Study, which spanned over twenty-five years, reviewed all the known factors in coronary heart disease. They concluded, "Over 50 percent of the variance in CHD death rates in twenty-five years were accounted for by the difference in mean serum cholesterol." A later follow-up stated, "Across cultures, cholesterol is linearly related to CHD mortality." The American Heart Association has consistently advised that the evidence linking elevated serum cholesterol to CHD is overwhelming. The legendary Framington Heart Study found that total cholesterol, triglycerides, HDL, and LDL levels taken together were the single most important determinant of heart disease.

Americans eat about 42 percent fat calories, and mostly all of them are from saturated animal fats. Substituting vegetable oils is simply lessening the harmful effects. Canola oil is a promotional fraud (seen any canola plants lately?), despite the hype and promotion by the so-called health food industry. Olive oil must be limited like any other vegetable oil. Corn, safflower, sunflower, and olive oils should be used in moderation. Soy oil tastes terrible unless it is highly refined. Sesame oil is very expensive, and toasted sesame oil is a condiment. Palm and coconut oils are meant for tropical peoples living in tropical climates. You should eat less than 20 percent fat calories, and these should be from vegetable sources, as well as seafood. This is very easy to do when you're not eating red meat, poultry, eggs, dairy products, fried foods, and junk foods. Less than 15 percent is even better.

TRIGLYCERIDES

At the University of Tor Vergata in Rome (*Acta Diabetologica* v. 40, 2003) people with metabolic syndrome were studied. The mean triglyceride level was a whopping 193. Again, the triglyceride count is the most meaningful blood lipid figure. The mean total cholesterol was 225. Their fasting blood sugar was 108, they were overweight, had high HDL and low LDL levels, hypertension, as well as high insulin. These people were given exercise capacity tests on a treadmill. They were all found to have diminished cardiovascular capacity, which indicates a much higher likelihood of heart and artery disease. People with metabolic syndrome die earlier and have a poorer quality of life, especially due to CHD conditions of all kinds. Triglycerides are the most important lipid indicator of blood sugar problems, and you must keep them under 100.

Sweets of all kinds, including honey and maple syrup, will raise your triglycerides levels, even on a low-fat diet. Vegans and ethical vegetarians are nearly always sugar addicts. They usually have elevated triglyceride levels, despite eating no saturated fats or animal foods at all. Fruit juice, dried fruit, stevia, honey, and agave are just as bad as white sugar.

Hydrogenated oils, often called trans fatty acids or partially hydrogenated oils, are the very worst fats. These are made by taking cheap oils (such as cottonseed) and forcing hydrogen gas into them, under extreme pressure and heat, with a platinum catalyst. Make sure you have none of these in your house, such as margarine or shortening. Margarine is not "better than butter" at all—it is even worse. You can buy non-hydrogenated, non-dairy spreads made of coconut and palm oils as a *temporary* transition (or occasional use) away from butter and margarine. Read the labels on any food you buy to make sure the word "hydrogenated" is not listed. Eating in fast food restaurants is almost guaranteed to get trans fats into your body. Eating in *any* restaurant is risky, since the types of oils and fats used in their foods are not mentioned on the menu. Studies around the world over the past few decades have proven repeatedly just how harmful these trans fats are, despite their popularity.

SUPPLEMENTS

If you are over the age of forty, you should basically be taking all the supplements listed in Chapter 6, "Effective Supplements" (see page 41). The most important cornerstone supplements are beta-sitosterol, flax oil, beta glucan, and soy isoflavones. There are other supplements you can take, like 3 g of guar gum, 3 g of fruit pectin (apple or grapefruit), 1,200 mg of lecithin, 3 g of gluco-mannon, and 3 g of sodium alginate. Please do not fall for such promotional scams as policosanol, red rice yeast, "modified" fruit pectin, and overdoses of niacin. Regardless of your age, you should be taking a complete mineral supplement with the twenty needed minerals in the required amounts. You can find one if you simply search the Internet under "mineral supplements." Look for one with all twenty of these vital elements in the biologically required amounts clearly stated on the label.

HORMONES

Doctors rarely understand the importance of our basic hormones on blood lipids. If you are over forty, you definitely need to test and balance your testosterone, DHEA, progesterone, pregnenolone, and melatonin, as well as your thyroid hormones T3 and T4. Women should also test their estradiol, estrone, and estriol. Please read Chapter 10, "Your Basic Hormones" (see page 81) for more information on this. Cholesterol is the biological source of all our sex hormones. The other hormones are pregnenolone, DHEA, testosterone, progesterone, androstenedione, estradiol, estrone, and estriol. Deficient or excessive hormone levels interfere with cholesterol metabolism. Doctors have no idea that our basic hormone levels strongly affect our cholesterol and triglyceride levels, so they don't bother to test hormone levels in people with high blood fats.

In 2002, the Mississippi Regional Cancer Center published a study titled, "Hypercholesteremia Treatment: A New Hypothesis" (*Medical Hypotheses* v. 59, 2002). These progressive doctors treated people with high cholesterol and triglycerides by balancing their basic endocrine levels. They used bioidentical hormones. They tested their levels and then appropriately prescribed DHEA, testosterone, T3, T4, pregnenolone, progesterone, estradiol, estrone, estriol, and cortisone (cortisol). These doctors realized that our entire endocrine system must be in balance, and that all our hormones work together in concert, as a team in harmony. We need more such progressive clinicians, as well as more such enlightening studies. This was a stunning study by first-rate physicians!

CONCLUSION

Lipids are one of the influences that affect the risk of coronary heart disease. The two main forms of lipids are cholesterol and triglycerides. Keeping your blood fats low will go a long way in keeping you healthy and enabling you to live a long, enjoyable life. Heart and artery disease is the major cause of mortality around the world by far. Cholesterol and triglycerides are the most accurate indicators of CHD health, and heart attacks are a primary cause of death in diabetic patients.

13. Obesity

Obesity is a disease characterized by an excess of body fat, and it is second in importance only to diet as a factor in blood sugar problems. The contributory causes of obesity include a range of factors, such as overconsumption, the type of food eaten, lack of exercise, and lifestyle. No one disputes the influence of being overweight. A whopping 80 percent of type 2 diabetics are overweight! Half of American adults are overweight or obese, and people in other countries are quickly following our path. With affluence comes obesity and high rates of all types of disease. One out of every two people in developed countries is overweight or obese, and that statistic continues to grow. And while newly developing countries' populations have traditionally been underweight, those countries that have introduced our Western diets into their societies have seen a triple increase in their rates of obesity. We will therefore spend our time discussing how to realistically lose weight and stay slim.

The US Department of Health and Human Services found that losing a mere 7 percent of body weight resulted in more than a 50-percent reduction in the incidence of adult-onset (type 2) diabetes. For a 200-pound person this is a mere 14 pounds. Just a one-fifteenth drop! Being overweight has almost every negative effect on your health imaginable. Obesity is clinically associated with high insulin, high glucose, hypertension, high cholesterol, high triglycerides, increased insulin resistance, high CRP levels, high homocysteine levels, high uric acid, high leptin, and low antioxidant levels. Add to this list high cardiovascular disease rates, early death, poor quality of life, increased oxidative stress and free radicals, high cancer rates of most types, lowered immunity, increased inflammation, and higher rates of depression, as well as other psychological problems. The only positive factor, ironically, is stronger bones in some people due to increased body mass index (BMI).

OBESITY IN CHILDREN

It is only in the last two decades that we have seen obesity affect American children and adolescents, especially Latin, African, and Asian Americans, and Amerindians. Type 1 and type 2 diabetes, insulin resistance, hyperinsulinemia, hypoglycemia, hypertension, high cholesterol and triglycerides, are all alarmingly increasing in these overweight children. One in three American children will grow up diabetic. Type 1-diabetes used to be called "childhood-onset diabetes," and type 2, "adult-onset." Commonly, children are now coming down with type 2 diabetes. The distinction is blurring. One important factor here is the public (which are really government schools and not "public" institutions) school lunch programs. Children are fed high-fat, high-sugar, and heavily refined foods with little nutrition. Dairy products and other food subsidy programs are promoted. Private and parochial schools don't do much better. Children also commonly eat meals in fast food restaurants. The food at home isn't much healthier either.

HOW OBESITY AFFECTS DIABETES

The American Diabetes Association, the North American Association for the Study of Obesity, and the American Society for Clinical Nutrition recently issued the statement (*American Journal of Clinical Nutrition* v. 80, 2004), "Weight management through lifestyle modification [is essential] for the prevention and management of type 2 diabetes. Overweight and obesity are important risk factors for type 2 diabetes. The marked increase in the prevalence of overweight and obesity is presumably responsible for the recent increase in type 2 diabetes. Lifestyle modification aimed at reducing energy intake and increasing physical activity is the principal therapy for overweight and obese patients with type 2 diabetes. The prevalence of diabetes in the United States continues to rise by epidemic proportions. This increase parallels the rising rates of obesity and overweight observed over the last decade. Indeed, as BMI (Body Mass Index) increases, the risk of developing type 2 diabetes increases in a dose-dependent manner. The prevalence of type 2 diabetes in obese adults is three to seven times that in normal weight adults. Those with a BMI greater than 35 are twenty times as likely to develop diabetes as those with a BMI between 18.5 and 24.9. In addition, weight gain during adulthood is directly correlated with an increased risk of type 2 diabetes. Obesity also complicates the management of type 2 diabetes by increasing insulin resistance and blood glucose concentrations. Obesity is an independent risk factor for dyslipidemia, hypertension, and CHD, and thus increases the risk of cardiovascular complications and cardiovascular mortality in patients with type 2 diabetes. Weight loss is an important goal for overweight and obese persons, particularly those with type 2 diabetes, because it improves glycemic control. Moderate weight loss (5 percent of body weight) can improve insulin action, decrease fasting blood glucose concentrations, and reduce the need for diabetes medications. Moreover, improvements in fasting blood glucose are directly related to the relative amount of weight loss."

MAINTAINING A HEALTHY WEIGHT

Want clinical proof from Cornell University (*American Journal of Clinical Nutrition* v. 46, 1987) that you can literally eat all you want, lose weight, and never be hungry? Women were allowed to eat all the whole natural foods they wanted, as long as they had 20 percent or less fat calories. They could eat 24 hours a day! In only 30 days, they lost considerable weight just by eating foods lower in fat. The ones who ate the 30 percent fat diet lost no weight. Your fat calorie intake must be under 20 percent, although 15 percent is better. Again, the average American eats about 42 percent fat calories, and most of these are saturated animal fats. There are many more similar published clinical studies showing the very same results.

Realistically, how do you lose weight, stay slim, never be hungry, and enjoy your food? Making better food choices is the key here. Along with making better food choices, there are many proven natural supplements to take that keep your metabolism at peak potential. Natural hormone balance is basic here. Lastly, regular exercise is always a part of maintaining normal weight.

The chart below shows how many pounds of each of the following foods you would have to eat in order to get 2,500 calories. For example, you could eat 0.9 pounds of peanuts or almost 12 pounds of grapes.

To obtain approximately 2,500 calories, you would have to eat the following foods (measured in pounds):

apples	9.4	cantaloupe	18.2
avocado	3.3	carrots	13.0
bananas	6.4	cauliflower	20.2
beans, green	21.9	celery	32.8
beans, navy	4.8	cheese	1.5
beans, pinto	5.3	chicken	3.2
beef, sirloin	1.2	chips, corn	2.0
blueberries	8.8	chips, potato	1.8
butter	0.8	chocolate	1.0
cabbage	22.8	chuck steak	1.4

corn	6.5		potatoes	9.6
cucumbers	32.8		rice, brown	5.1
eggs	3.4		salmon	3.9
French fries	1.7		shrimp	4.8
grapes	11.9		soymilk	10.1
ham	2.1		spinach	21.0
honey	1.8		squash	28.8
lamb chops	2.2		sugar, white	1.5
lettuce	39.0		sweet potato	5.4
mangos	8.3		turkey	2.1
oatmeal	6.0		vegetable oil	0.6
onions	14.8		walnuts	0.9
oranges	15.6		whole wheat bread	4.0
peanuts	0.9		whole wheat pasta	3.1

It's obvious that meat, poultry, eggs (50 percent fat calories), and dairy products are basically highest in fat and, therefore, highest in calories. Whole grains and beans are very filling, yet low in fat and calories. Vegetables and fruits are the lowest of all. You can eat all you want, never be hungry, and stay slim and trim just by choosing healthier, low-fat foods to eat.

We need only two meals a day. The less you eat the better. Americans eat twice the amount of calories they need. Don't eat out. Take your lunch to work. A man needs only about 1,800 calories a day, and a woman needs only about 1,200 calories. Don't eat breakfast, and you'll have more time in the morning. Or you can eat breakfast and supper, and skip lunch. You'll save time, money, and energy by not eating three times a day. Soon this will feel very natural to you, and you won't want to eat three meals a day anymore. You may not be able to fast for more than eight or twelve hours until you are well. When you are well, you should fast every week for twenty-four hours on water, from dinner to dinner.

CONCLUSION

As this chapter has shown, a link exists between obesity and diabetes. It is becoming clear that the conveniences that we are presented with today lead to less physical activity, high-fat and high-energy diets, and convenient foods, which lead to being overweight. This excess weight places an extra stress on our bodies, resulting in conditions that lead to becoming diabetic.

14. Exercise Is Essential

So you have been told that you have diabetes. You can sit on your rear, take medications, and hope for the best, or you can do something that costs nothing, is easy to do, and has no dangerous side effects. What is it? Exercise regularly. You can do resistance or aerobic exercise, or both, but you must exercise regularly. There is no way around this! No matter how well you eat, how many proven supplements you take, and how well you balance your endocrine hormone system, you still need to exercise to cure diabetes and similar blood sugar conditions. The literature is overwhelmingly clear on this. Exercise burns off that blood sugar. Since researchers around the world agree on this, we won't bother to cite the journals for the studies mentioned.

WALKING

Walking is probably the best and single most enjoyable exercise of all. It is a widely recommended form of physical activity for people who have been diagnosed with diabetes. A simple half-hour brisk walk of two miles a day is all you really need. Of course, two brisk half-hour walks, totaling four miles a day, would be *twice* as good. Besides helping you slim down, walking is effective at controlling the glucose levels in your blood, as well as your blood pressure.

111

AEROBIC EXERCISE

Aerobic exercise works to lower your blood sugar. This steady exercise performed over a period of time makes the heart and lungs stronger, the body uses more oxygen, and it uses up blood sugar. An aerobic workout may include jogging, swimming, dancing, or bicycling.

RESISTANCE EXERCISE

Resistance exercise is just as good as aerobic exercise here, and the combination of *both* resistance and aerobic would be the ideal. Doing both resistance and aerobic activity is the very best program you can do. Resistance exercise is also known as strength training. Basically, there are three different ways to do your resistance workout: on a weight machine, using free weights, and performing calisthenics, such as sit-ups and chin-ups.

Tai chi just isn't realistically going to help you here, as it is extremely hard to learn and doesn't get your blood flowing. Gym membership is very inexpensive and a wonderful investment. When you begin any kind of exercise program, warm up before you start and cool down at the end. Over time, you can steadily increase the length and intensity of the workout.

THE SCIENCE BEHIND THE FACTS

At the University of Perugia in Italy, a fine article was published called, "Make Your Diabetic Patients Walk." They found that the more walking the patients did, the more they improved. Blood pressure fell, cholesterol and triglyceride levels fell, they lost weight, their waist measurement was smaller, and fasting glucose levels were lowered, with no other lifestyle changes. Just brisk walking two or more miles a day gave dramatic results.

At the renowned Harvard Medical School two heavily referenced reviews were done on exercise and type 2 diabetes. Regular physical exercise proved to be vital for both the prevention and treatment of type 2 diabetes. Regular physical exercise with dietary restrictions increased energy expenditure. This leads to decreased body weight, increased insulin sensitivity, improved long-term glycemic control and lipid profiles, lower blood pressure, and increased cardiovascular fitness.

Two very good studies were done at the University of Barcelona, in Spain. Both type 1 and 2 diabetics exercised regularly for three months. Their physical fitness and aerobic capacity improved of course. Their insulin requirements were reduced, their waist measurement shrank, their blood pressure fell, Lp(a) (lipoprotein) levels fell, and their blood lipid profile improved. All this occurred with no change in diet or supplements, just regular exercise. You must exercise to normalize blood sugar and insulin.

Diabetes is an epidemic in Finland, as it is in all European countries. At the National Public Health Institute, it was shown that both resistance and aerobic exercise are effective in normalizing blood sugar metabolism in two separate studies. The role of physical activity in the prevention of NIDDM is of utmost importance. Both circuit-type resistance training and aerobic endurance exercise had beneficial effects in subjects with impaired glucose tolerance. The University of Kuopio and Helsinki University found that the same effects occurred in type 1 diabetics.

It is difficult to treat obese diabetics for many reasons. Overweight women at the University of Texas performed regular exercise. This exercise training resulted in significant weight loss, and lowered the insulin response to an oral glucose load (i.e. improved insulin sensitivity). Remember, this was done with no change in diet. Exercise alone results in meaningful weight loss. If the women had been given a low-fat, whole-grain-based diet, and a full spectrum of supplements and minerals, they would have further improved insulin response and lost even more weight.

Postmenopausal women, especially obese ones, in America can be difficult to treat because they usually have multiple health conditions. At the University of Maryland in Baltimore, obese postmenopausal women (aged fifty to sixty-five) performed resistance training (RT) exercise regularly for a few months. The gained strength, lost weight, lowered their body fat percent, and improved their insulin sensitivity. The conclusion was that RT has the potential to ameliorate, and even prevent, the development of insulin resistance and reduce the risk of glucose intolerance, as well as NIDDM, in postmenopausal women. Just simple exercise accomplished this, with no changes in diet or lifestyle.

At Kansai Denryoku Hospital in Japan, two separate studies of type 2 diabetics were done. In the first study, only exercise was used. Their insulin sensitivity immediately improved, and their glucose and triglyceride levels both fell strongly. The researchers felt the lower trigylceride levels were the most important factor for the improvement of diabetes with exercise. In the second study, exercise was combined with a low-fat traditional Japanese-style diet. They concluded that short-term (7 days) low-intensity physical exercise combined with a traditional diet reduced serum triglycerides, insulin resistance, and fasting glucose levels. Only one week of exercise accomplished medical miracles. Just one week!

At Syracuse University, two separate studies using resistance, rather than aerobic, exercise were done. In the first study resistance exercise reduced glucose levels in type 2 female diabetics. They found resistance exercise offered an alternative to aerobic exercise for improving glucose control in diabetic patients. To realize optimal glucose control benefits, you must follow a regular schedule that includes daily exercise. In the second study, male and female diabetics got the same results from exercising, with no other treatments or lifestyle changes.

Researchers at the University of Western Australia did four studies. They used resistance (strength training) exercise for just thirty minutes a day, three times a week—ninety minutes a week—and found this provided a practical addition to lifestyle management of type 2 diabetes in only eight weeks. Resistance exercise (circuit training) was found to be an effective method that improved functional capacity, lean body mass, strength, and glycemic control of patients. One of the studies found that moderate exercise and a diet (including fish) high in omega-3 fatty acids improved various diagnostic factors for type 2 diabetes. Another study lowered glucose by 13 percent and insulin by 20 percent with just mild exercise. At St. Vincent's Hosptial in Sydney, type 1 diabetics improved their health with just forty-five minutes of cycling a day. Again, feeding whole complex carbohydrates prior to exercise prevented hypoglycemia.

At the famous Brigham and Women's Hospital in Boston, a massive twenty-six page review with 168 references was done on exercise in both type 1 and 2 diabetics. There is no doubt that regular exercise has numerous benefits for blood sugar conditions. Physical exercise is an important adjunct in the treatment of both NIDDM and IDDM (insulin-dependent diabetes mellitus). There is now extensive epidemiological evidence demonstrating that long-term physical exercise can significantly reduce the risk of developing NIDDM. Glucose uptake, glucose control, insulin sensitivity, GLUT4 (a marker for glucose uptake) is raised, and glucose transport are all improved. This is the most extensive published review ever done, and it is simply inarguable that exercise is essential when it comes to managing and preventing blood sugar disorders.

CONCLUSION

Regular exercise is important for everyone, but it is especially important if you have diabetes. When you have blood sugar dysmetabolism of any kind, you must get regular exercise. Having an exercise regimen helps control the amount of sugar in the blood and it also burns off excess calories and fat to help you achieve a desirable healthy weight. Maintaining a healthy weight is crucial in taking care of your diabetes. It also lowers your risk of coronary heart disease, which is common in people who have diabetes. Ideally, you will do both resistance and aerobic exercise, but it just doesn't matter as long you do one or the other. You'll live longer and live better this way.

Seven Steps to Natural Health

The following steps are of vital importance if you want to live a long and healthy life. With these seven steps you can cure "incurable" illnesses like cancer, diabetes, heart disease, and others naturally without drugs, surgery, or chemotherapy. These are seven vital steps to take if you want optimum health and a long life. Do your best to do all of them. The only step to add would be prayer or meditation.

1. Maintain an American macrobiotic whole grain-based diet. Diet is the most crucial factor in achieving good health. Diet cures disease. Everything else is secondary.

2. Take proven supplements to enhance the effects of your diet. There are only about twenty scientifically recommended for those over forty, and eight for those under forty.

3. Balance your hormone levels. The fourteen basic hormones are listed in Chapter 10 (see page 81), and you can easily (and inexpensively) measure your hormone levels from the comfort of your own home.

4. Exercise regularly, even if it is just a half hour of walking a day. Exercise is vital, and it is best to have a balanced workout of aerobic or resistance training.

5. Fasting is the most powerful healing method known to man. Fast one day a week. Drink only water from dinner to dinner. Join our monthly Young Again two-day fast—the fasting calendar is at www.YoungAgain.org during the last weekend of every month.

6. Do not take prescription drugs, except *temporary* antibiotics or pain medication during an emergency. (Of course, there are rare exceptions such as insulin for type 1 diabetics, who have no operant pancreas.)

7. Limit or end any bad habits such as drinking alcohol or coffee, using recreational drugs, and eating desserts. You don't have to be a saint, but you do need to be sincere.

Resources

Recommended Reading

Book of Macrobiotics by Michio Kushi, Japan Publications, Inc., 1986

Eat More, Weigh Less by Dean Ornish, MD, Quill. 2001

Eat Right, Live Longer: Using the Natural Power of Foods to Age-Proof Your Body by Neal Barnard, MD, Harmony Books, 1998

Food for Life: How the New four Food Groups Can Save Your Life by Neal Barnard, MD, Three Rivers Press, 1994

Get Healthy Now! A Complete Guide to Prevention, Treatment and Healthy Living, by Gary Null, PhD, Seven Stories Press, 1999

The Good Carbohydrate Revolution: A Proven Program for Low-Maintenance Weight Loss and Optimum Health by Terry Shintani, MD, JD, MPH, Pocket Books, 2003

The Hawaii Diet by Terry Shintani, MD, JD, MPH, Pocket Books, 1999

Live Longer, Live Better by Neal Barnard, MD, Book Publishing Company (TN), 1997 (audio)

Macrobiotic Diet by Michio Kushi and Aveline Kushi, Japan Publications, Inc.,1993

Macrobiotic Way by Michio Kushi, Penguin Group, Inc., 2004

Macrobiotics for Dummies by Verne Verona, Wiley Publishing, Inc.,2009

Macrobiotics for Life by Simon Brown, North Atlantic Books, 2009

Program for Reversing Heart Disease by Dean Ornish, MD, Ballantine Books, 1996

The 7 Steps to Perfect Health by Gary Null, PhD, iBooks, 2001

Stop the Insanity by Susan Powter, Pocket Books, 1993

Turn Off the Fat Genes: The Revolutionary Guide to Losing Weight by Neal Barnard, MD, Harmony Books, 2001

The Vegetarian Handbook: Eating Right for Total Health, Gary Null, PhD, St. Martin's Press, 1996

Zen Macrobiotics by George Ohsawa, George Ohsawa Macrobiotic Foundation, 1995

About the Author

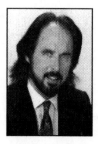

Roger Mason is an internationally known research chemist who studies natural health and longevity. He has written ten different unique and cutting edge books about his findings. He sold Beta Prostate® in 2011, walked away from radio and TV, and formed a charitable trust. He lives with his wife and dog in Wilmington, NC, where they run Young Again Products. You can get his free weekly newsletter, read his books, and his 300 articles for free at www.youngagain.org.

Index